THE CODE OF A HEALTHY MIND

DISCOVER THE HEALTH MINDSET AND START
LIVING YOUR HEALTHIEST AND HAPPIEST LIFE

TATIANA M. KEAY

Copyright © 2021 by Tatiana Keay

All rights reserved.

No part of this book may be reproduced in any form or by any electronic or mechanical means, including information storage and retrieval systems, without written permission from the author, except for the use of brief quotations in a book review.

ISBN: 9798535727851

For my Babushka and Dedushka

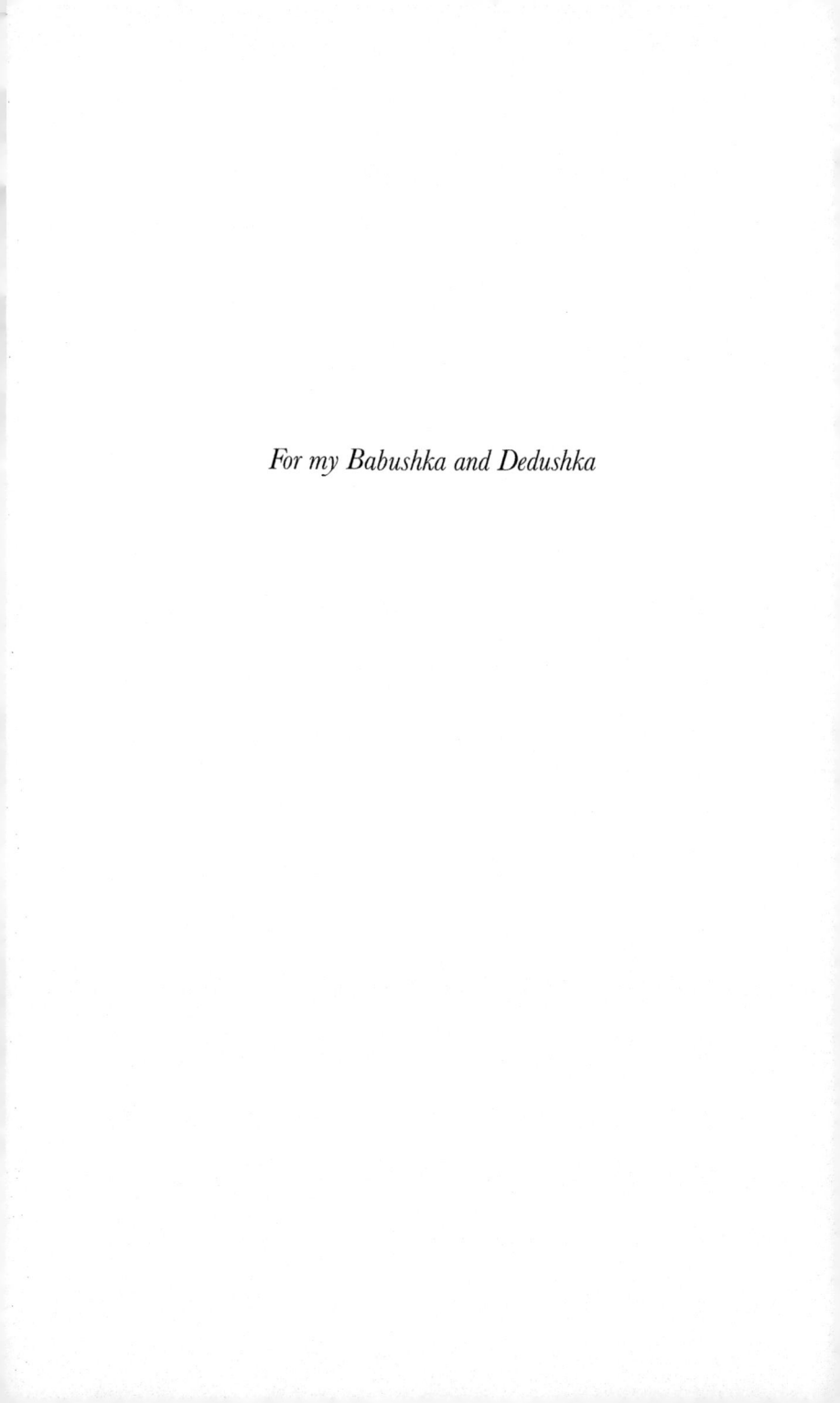

CONTENTS

Introduction	vii
1. Belief Systems	1
2. The Dieter's Mindset	17
3. The Health Mindset	29
4. Awareness	47
5. Rewiring Your Beliefs	59
6. Rewrite Your Definition of Health	78
7. Eating Well	100
8. Trust Your Body Temple	114
9. The Never-Ending Story	127
Next Steps for YOUR Health Journey	147
Acknowledgments	149
Notes	153

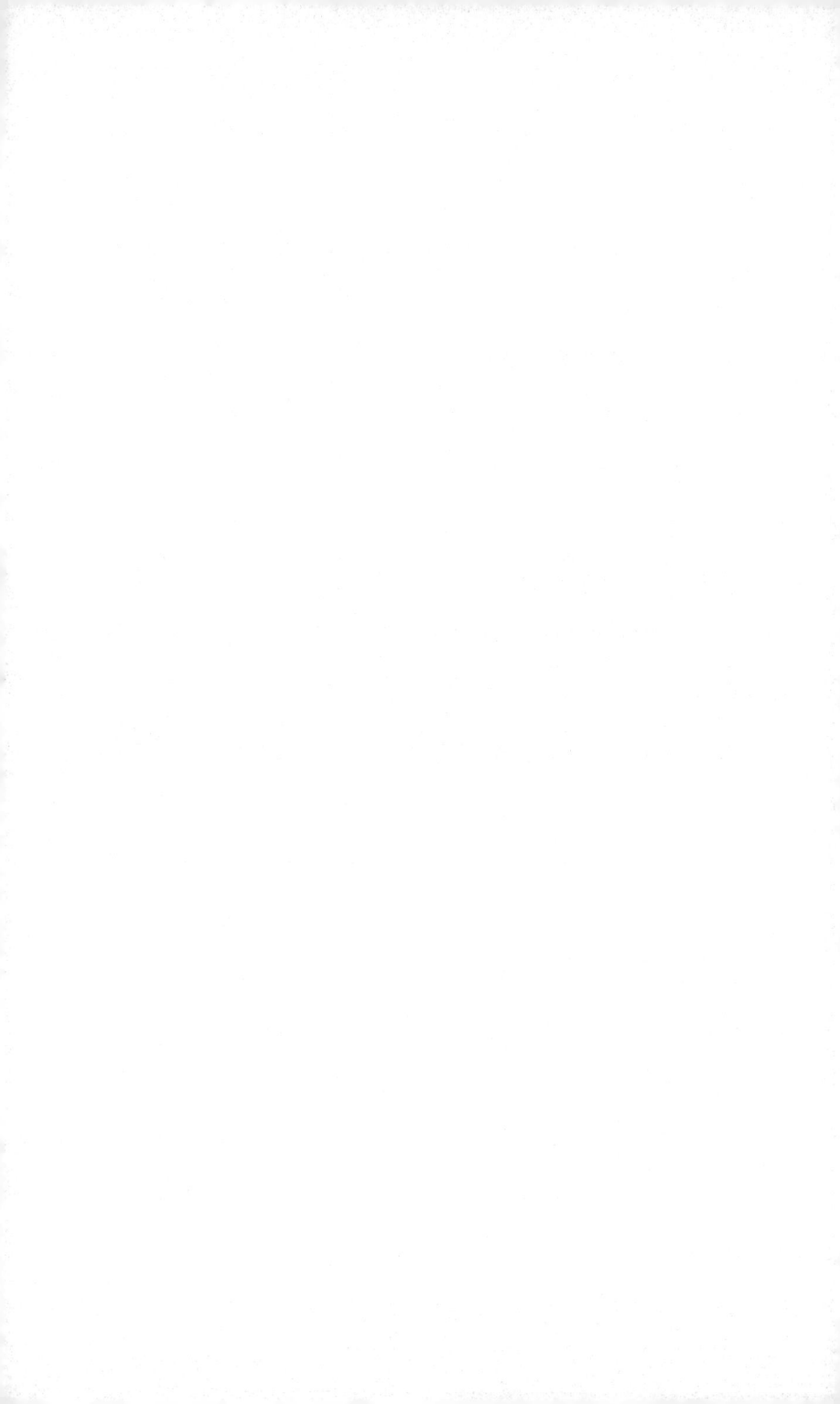

INTRODUCTION

After a deep breath, I open the door and call the patient's name. She stands up from her seat and gathers her things on the other side of the lobby. As she walks through the open door, I greet her with a smile. I ask her to step on the scale as the door closes gently behind me. After jotting down the number on the scale, I lead her back to the room I use for my nutrition consultations. I invite her to sit and ask why she came to see me today. She starts the familiar story I've heard so many times before.

I've struggled with my weight for a very long time. I've tried everything. I've counted my calories, been following the Weight Watchers program to a tee, and I'm trying to avoid bad foods. I've been able to lose weight in the past many times, but this time, I don't know what I'm doing wrong.

I observe the despair in her eyes as I listen

intently. I understand, so I nod. I've experienced it too before: desperation to lose weight. I know the prison she is living in. And at that moment, there's nothing more I desire in life than to help her. So, I begin my investigation. What are her favorite foods? What times does she eat? What beverages does she drink? What is her physical activity level? And many more questions. I immerse myself in her lifestyle as if it were my own, on the lookout for the red flags.

Occasionally, I break eye contact and type away ferociously on my outdated work laptop. Plenty of red squiggly lines appear in my chart note as I try to keep up while she tells me about what she ate this weekend. By the time she has completed her story, I have an incoherent document only I can understand.

A feeling of relief enters my body when I locate the problem source. I relax, waiting patiently for my turn to speak. I ask for her permission to provide feedback. Most patients are ready to hear my recommendations. Unfortunately, a small percentage is not (these patients go on to beg for weight loss medications). Luckily, she was one of the many who welcomed my feedback with hope and optimism.

Together, we create a realistic health plan to support her weight loss journey. After answering any remaining questions, I walk her out of the exam room, back to the lobby. I observe her energy as she walks out. She already appears much freer and less burdened. I know there's a lot of work to do. Not the "work" of eating more vegetables or decreasing sugar intake—but mindset work.

You see, like many of my prior patients who sat in the same chair in that same exam room, she too had a dieter's mindset. A mindset that causes many women to despise their one and only amazing body. An attitude that destroys a wonderful part of life: eating and sharing delicious meals with the ones you love. A philosophy that distracts you from the joy of living in the present moment.

The dieter's mindset is the prison you don't realize you're in until you've escaped. It's a prison constructed by your external environment: the people who raised you, teachers, friends, and the media. It's not their fault, though, because they are in their own cages. Blame is just another unfortunate thing we've been taught to do.

I'm not afraid to admit that I have struggled with an unhealthy perspective about food and my body in the past. I grew up as a shy little girl who ate more like a bird than a growing child to the point where everyone thought my younger sister was older than I was. Growing up, my family was incredibly health-conscious, which I now know is a luxury, but at the time, it felt more like a punishment. My dad was controlling about the sort of foods that my family ate, and when the first health food store opened near our home, he was ecstatic. He would insist on only organic food and absolutely nothing processed. While other kids would have Oreos or fruit punch tucked into their elementary school lunches, I had carrots and water with a sandwich made with Ezekiel bread. We hardly ever indulged in treats or processed food—let alone keep anything like that in the house.

Once I was in high school, I had more autonomy. I could make my own choices as far as my diet went, and I started eating all the things I wanted—regardless of how healthy or unhealthy my family might deem it. I started buying whatever I wanted from the lunch bar, which was usually Hot Cheetos and cream cheese. I would drive through Del Taco with my friends after tennis practice and order some soft chicken tacos. When I was home, I only remember eating bowls of cereal, lost in the sweet forbidden crunch, and drinking every drop of milk.

I wasn't eating to be healthy. I didn't eat to fuel my body for tennis practice or to ensure I was clear-headed during school. I ate whatever I wanted because I could. After tennis season was over, I continued to eat as if I worked out two hours per day. And it began to show itself physically. It was like I woke up one morning to a completely different body than I remembered having only the day before. No one prepared me for the maturing body transformation every girl goes through. I thought I was always going to be skin and bones.

This was my initiation into the dieting world. The awareness of having bigger thighs triggered the cycle of restrictive dieting and overeating. I would cut my calories and avoid my favorite foods, which resulted in feelings of deprivation. And it wasn't long before I binge ate multiple bowls of cereal. For years, my weight crept up during the winter seasons and dropped back down during summertime. I was stuck on a pendulum, swinging from one extreme to another. I never learned the middle road; how to fuel myself with whole foods but still allow myself the flexibility to enjoy less nutritious foods.

I was dieting until I started my nutrition program, and this is when my beliefs started to unconsciously shift. Through my studies as a dietitian, I learned more about how food interacts with your body and your body interacts with food. Dietitian school rewired how I perceived "dieting," and my relationship with food began to heal. For the first time, I entered a space that was somewhere between eating nutritious foods, splurging, and dieting. I began cultivating an empowered relationship with food that allowed me freedom, joy, and health. Now I have fully experienced life without living by the rules of diet culture.

For most of those years I struggled, I thought I was to blame for my body image issues and poor eating behaviors. I thought it was just the way things are. I know you've picked up this book because you've felt this way too. Every diet book you've tried before seems to be spewing something different. One book tells you to stop eating carbs, yet another book tells you to eat carbs, but only certain kinds and at certain times of the day, while another book tells you why you shouldn't have anything with lectins. You've tried it all before, but no diet book has been able to give you the freedom, health, and happiness that was pictured on the cover. *Sure*, you think, *it worked for her because she's HER. She doesn't know what it's like.* When you're through with a diet, you often feel worse about yourself than when you started and five feet further away from your initial goal. It's overwhelming for anyone to navigate the health and wellness field, let alone someone who's just trying to get their health under control to live a more energized and vibrant life.

By the time you finish this book and do the necessary internal work, I hope you will finally feel at home in your body. You will have the confidence, happiness, health, and well-being you once thought was impossible. In addition, you will have a healthy relationship with food and eating, which will make up part of the foundation of healthy habits for the rest of your life.

Together, we're going to examine the root cause of your unwanted and unhealthful eating behaviors; why you continue to struggle with your health despite having a multitude of "answers" at your fingertips. I will walk you through the same process I have personally coached hundreds of my patients through. I am going to show you how to rewire your brain to finally experience success with nutrition, create your own picture of health, and establish a new set of empowering beliefs to match it. This book is hopefully just the start for you on your unique health journey but is sure to radically transform your relationship with your body and with food.

It is possible to rewire your brain so you can live your happiest and healthiest life without restriction and shame. If you are finally ready to take responsibility for your health and mindset, you are in the right place. If you are prepared to drop the struggle and make nutrition easier, this path is yours.

The single decision to take responsibility for your own life is powerful enough to break the cycle. In an attempt to help you transform into your healthiest self, I kindly suggest that you keep an open mind. If we are going to get you from point A to point B successfully, we will have to make some changes. I'll hand over the key, but you are the one that must unlock the chains. And maybe one day, you'll wake up and realize you have the body you've dreamed about. Your happier, healthier life is waiting for you as soon as you're ready to awaken to it.

1

BELIEF SYSTEMS

It was the summer before my nineteenth birthday when I made the life-altering decision that changed my life trajectory. After years of gossiping and making bad life choices, I had enough toxicity. I grabbed a black dry erase marker and wrote "*I am good*" in clear lettering on my mirror. I took a step back and read each word slowly, noticing my blurry bleach blonde reflection. The glimpse of myself and the word *good* shifted something in my mind. A new brain connection was created, and I was forever changed that afternoon.

Choosing to be a better person expanded my consciousness in a way I didn't know existed. I didn't know I could take responsibility for my life. Sometimes, an increase in awareness happens intentionally, and at other times, it's accidental. Either way, this expansion of consciousness occurs many times throughout our lives. Some people are more aware than others, and some never fully awaken. When we step up and choose, accept, or let go of what happens in our life, we live consciously.

There's a picture that pops into my head whenever I think about the vastness of our minds. In one of my grade school classrooms, there hung a poster of an iceberg. You've probably seen it before because the psychologist Freud used it as a representation of human consciousness. The tip of the iceberg that exists on top of the water exemplifies the conscious mind. It's visible, candid, and easy to understand. Beneath the water, though, exists the grander part of the iceberg. This more significant chunk of ice represents unconscious beliefs and unseen thoughts: the subconscious mind.

The subconscious mind is the part of us that deceives us. This is where your programming from childhood is stored. It's where negative thoughts run free and untamed without your knowing. It's where painful memories are stored, locked away from being remembered until accidentally triggered to escape into your awareness. It's where hard lessons are stowed, like when you allowed yourself to be vulnerable with someone you trusted, only to be betrayed. While there is a lot of darkness beneath the water, it's also where hidden gems are found. Your unique gifts, truths, and desires are weaved throughout the uncomfortable fragments of the subconscious mind.

Most of our belief systems are found deep within the subconscious mind. Belief systems are a set of rules or principles which code our life. They are the foundation of how you view the world. Different beliefs will shift your perspective. Simply put, this internal framework creates your external reality.

Our beliefs are woven into everything we do and everything we touch. Even though beliefs infiltrate every aspect of our life, we never sit down to investigate them, usually because people equate "beliefs" with religion; however, believing in something goes far beyond religion. This may be a hard pill to swallow at first, but most of the ideas you hold about yourself and the world aren't even your own beliefs. These beliefs are the thoughts and feelings of others you unconsciously accept as truth. Understanding your belief systems is essential in the conversation about health. Whether you're aware of it or not, your beliefs hinder you from attaining health and happiness. The good news is beliefs themselves are entirely subjective. Beliefs can be emitted, rewritten, or enhanced with conscious practice and effort.

That summer afternoon, I laughed when I realized I could take responsibility for my life and become whoever I wanted. Thank goodness my innate desire to be good caught my awareness. Because this one decision rewrote my mental code and impacted my life for the better. The very moment you take responsibility for your life is when the magic begins to seep in. Within months, I cultivated meaningful relationships, got promoted to manager at work, strengthened my body, met the love of my life, and experienced unconditional love.

While I can't tell you the exact meaning of life, I know life is not meant to be lived passively in a state of unwellness. You were not put here on this little rock, circling a little sun, in an incomprehensibly massive universe to feel unhappy or unwell. As you regain control of the pen writing your life story, we will rewrite the belief systems that do not serve and support your health journey.

When I think about this journey of expanding awareness and rewriting belief systems, I like to think about Plato's story, *Allegory of the Cave*. In this story, a group of prisoners was born and raised in a dark cave. In this cave, the prisoners were chained and forced to stare at the wall in front of them. A small fire behind them burned day and night, and those traveling on the walkway above them produced shadows on the wall. The prisoners made up little stories for the shapes that passed by. Since the cave and shadows were all the prisoners knew, they believed this was the extent of the world. They thought that everyone else must live in a dimly lit cave and experience the world in the form of shadows.

One day, a prisoner escaped. He ran from the cave and out into the daylight, where he was blinded by the sun. After his eyes were able to adjust, the world around him slammed into focus. The man saw green grass and a blue sky for the first time ever. He ran his hands across tree bark and dipped his toes into the nearby stream. He couldn't believe this reality existed.

He ended up getting captured and retaken prisoner, but he couldn't forget what he just experienced. Before leaving the cave, he believed all that existed in the world were shadows on a cave wall; he didn't know anything more. But now, returning to the cave, he knew a whole other world existed beyond the walls, full of three-dimensional objects and color. He tried to explain what he experienced to the other prisoners, but he didn't have the words to describe it. They thought maybe he had lost his mind, and so, they continued to watch the shadows on the walls.

This story boils down to an increase in consciousness. The temporarily freed prisoner became aware of his flawed, limiting beliefs when he experienced life outside his cave. With his discovery of color and nature, his faulty beliefs were rewritten to represent something that was now true for him. Like the prisoners in the cave, most of us are entirely unaware of our beliefs until we are confronted with another way of thinking. We live in the dark because that's what everyone else seems to be doing. We accept that all our beliefs and thoughts are the truth, but most of the time, that couldn't be further from the case.

Beliefs are collections of thought patterns and can often be shared, validated, and integrated by a group of people. When you become aware that beliefs are fluid, subjective, and pervasive, examine them to ensure your beliefs serve your purpose. You want a belief system that encourages you to be a good person and paves a path towards your dreams. Empowering beliefs are not meant to keep you small and stuck where you are right now, or worse, spiraling down further into a life you don't wish for. When you begin to shine a light on your previously programmed beliefs, you may find some codes which are not serving you or your health. Before we get into empowering and disempowering beliefs, it is important to understand where beliefs come from and how your beliefs create your reality.

If you've never paused to question where your beliefs come from, you're not alone. Most people haven't given their beliefs a second thought, putting blind faith in them. But they don't just appear in your head out of nowhere. Your beliefs about everything—from money, relationships, and success to love and happiness—were created by *something*. Most of our beliefs were programmed by familial rules and traditions, some entirely made up like fairy tales. And a boatload of our ideas originates from the current culturescape around us.

I like the word *culturescape* because it's a great representation of the bubble we live in. The term culturescape was coined by Vishen Lakhiani in his book, *The Code of the Extraordinary Mind*, and is described as the bullsh*t rules people live by.[1] The culturescape you are born into determines the sorts of limiting beliefs you develop. And trust me, we all adopt limiting beliefs along the road to adulthood.

As children, we are told by adults that things are the way they are, and that is the end of it. We believe adults when they tell us stories about a fat man coming down the chimney to deliver us presents. Or the fairy who collects teeth in exchange for money. And so, we also believe them when they say things like *money is the root of all evil*, or *no one will love me because I'm fat*. Throughout our lives, we unconsciously invest our faith into beliefs that might not even be true, and unfortunately, beliefs that certainly do not serve us. There is no real way to avoid this programming as children. And as you get older, you are still surrounded by the culturescape, which implicitly impacts everything you do. It is so subtle that you probably haven't even noticed all the indoctrination that's occurred throughout your whole life.

The human brain likes to operate with the most ease and efficiency possible. We call this phenomenon the path of least resistance. The brain works this way because it has critical jobs that all need to be performed simultaneously, like digesting your food and breathing. So, whichever way your brain can save energy and operate on autopilot, it will. That's why we tend to repeat the same behavior patterns (AKA habits) even when we know better or are actively trying to make a change. Most of your behaviors have been repeated throughout your life, whether or not you've been aware of them.

I've had plenty of patients that have tried making eating healthy a habit. They come into their first nutrition consultation explaining how they've been trying to avoid bad foods. They rationalize how they buy low-fat yogurt or avoid all desserts at parties. They try to avoid fruit "because of the sugar," even though they really love it. They justify why last weekend was "not good" because their husband, who doesn't care about eating healthy, bought a gallon of ice cream. And when it's in the house, it is impossible to have self-control. I've seen patient after patient who describes a behavior change attempt, but they just can't seem to stick with it. These patients try to create healthy habits by restricting foods they often love. However, during the process of saying no or counting calories or points, willpower gets exhausted—and the brain has limited energy for willpower. This forceful method of behavior change isn't sustainable for most people, which reverts people back to the way they were eating before.

We often think about changing our behavior first. We hope the expensive juice cleanse or thirty-day no sugar plan will finally be the thing that kickstarts our new healthy lifestyle. The issue I've come to understand is eating, drinking, and exercising are *behaviors*. And behaviors are superficial in the scheme of things. Therefore, people continue to fail in sustaining new habits. To change a behavior, we have to take three steps back to understand where it's coming from. First, one must go deeper into your psyche to determine who the heck is driving your life. If behaviors are superficial, then what's the root problem? Why do you do the things you do? *Why* do you want to eat sugary foods? *Why* do you really want to skip your workout today? What is driving your behaviors?

The fact is your emotions control your behaviors. And your emotions are simply a result of what's whirling around in that brain of yours: thoughts. Most of your thoughts are unconscious and automatic—thanks to your programmed belief system. So, behaviors are just the result of emotions, thoughts, and belief systems. And our good ol' belief system is the root cause.

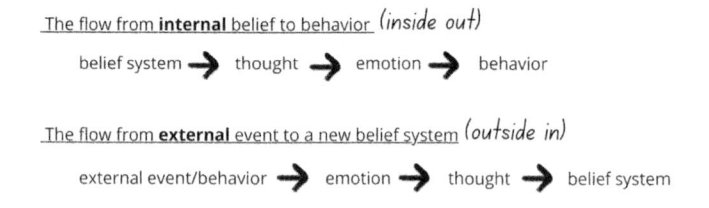

The flow from **internal** belief to behavior *(inside out)*
belief system ➜ thought ➜ emotion ➜ behavior

The flow from **external** event to a new belief system *(outside in)*
external event/behavior ➜ emotion ➜ thought ➜ belief system

Interestingly, the flow goes the opposite way when a new belief is created. When something happens in our external reality, it can spark an emotion within us. For example, when your mom told you to finish the food on your plate because it's not fair to starving little children, you may have felt the emotion of guilt and feeling sorry for them. That emotion triggers a thought. *I must never leave food on my plate.* When a thought is repeated enough times, it creates strong neural connections in the brain and eventually becomes a belief.

Our brain has over 6,000 thoughts a day, and most of them are the same, repetitive thoughts.[2] If you've been operating under the same beliefs since childhood, they are well wired into your system resulting in automatic habits you may not be aware of. These unconscious thoughts rule your emotions and, in turn, your behaviors themselves.

Take a patient of mine, for example. She came to see me because she had pre-diabetes and wanted to prevent it from getting any worse. During one of our sessions, she told me that she was teased by the other kids for being fat when she was in middle school. These kids verbalized that no one liked her, and she was gross. Even though she was just a kid at the time, and she was now an adult, her classmates' mean behavior struck a chord of inadequacy and shame within her. Her emotions triggered thoughts like: *Am I really fat? No one likes me because I'm fat, so fat must be a bad thing.* This message was reinforced by cultural expectations, society, the media, and even her own family throughout her life.

Because these thoughts were repeated every day for nearly 35 years, they took root in her mind as a belief system. All the struggles with eating a healthy diet came down to a negative belief about herself that she was unlovable because she was overweight. There was so much faith invested into this belief that it became normalized in her mind, so she never stopped to examine if it was true. This belief of not being good enough because she was overweight ended up hurting the quality of her life. Her mind was consumed with constant thoughts about food, her body, and weight. This led to unhealthful eating behaviors and years of poor body image and self-rejection. This belief that tied her worthiness as a human being to her weight was a *limiting* belief. This belief system operated under the surface in ways that negatively impacted her thoughts, emotions, and behavior. Therefore, it affected her whole life.

Limiting beliefs are the root cause of resistance and issues we experience in life. The more we become exposed to the world's arbitrary rules, the more limiting beliefs pile up in the dark corners of our minds. Limiting beliefs can extend to any area of your life: dating, friendships, family, food, exercise, money, career, success, spirituality. They are the reason you get stuck in the same patterns of behavior. This tends to leave us frustrated when we can't stick to any new habits or behaviors. For example, limiting beliefs are one of the main reasons why people have money problems. Despite their conscious desire and effort to make more money, the moment people have more of it, they lose it or spend it. Subconsciously a person might have a limiting belief that money is the root of all evil or that being rich makes you a bad person. If your unconscious beliefs are not in sync with your conscious desires, you will not make sustained progress towards your goals. So, before we start changing any eating behavior, we must uncover the root of the problem, which is your belief system. Limiting beliefs about your health are the most significant hurdle for you to overcome on your journey to well-being.

There are three different kinds of limiting beliefs to be aware of because each type will impact your thoughts, emotions, and behavior. The first type of limiting belief is about who you are. Limiting beliefs about who you are, what you're capable of, and how you're perceived by others will keep you small and stuck in one place. This results in the constant search for validation from other people and feeling like you are not good enough. Negative beliefs about yourself include thoughts like *I'm a loser*, *I'm a failure*, *I'm stupid*, or *I'm ugly*—and everything in between. These beliefs are disempowering, and until these beliefs are rewritten, you'll be stuck in the same behavior patterns.

The second type of limiting belief is the judgmental beliefs you have about other people. For example, if you believe your best friend is a kind and thoughtful person and she gives you a compliment, you might smile and thank her. But suppose a girl at work, who you believe is untrustworthy or manipulative, gives you the same compliment. In that case, you are less likely to smile and more inclined to wonder, *what does this chick want from me?* Believing that everyone is against you, cruel, or untrustworthy limits you from experiencing all the good and kindness that exists all around you in the world. The limiting beliefs we have about others get in the way of meaningful relationships, which is a vital component of well-being.

The third kind of limiting belief is beliefs about the world. This includes thinking that the fate of the world is doomed. Or that you can't be successful because of the government, or that the immigrants are taking your jobs. This kind of thinking leaves you with a victim mentality. It ultimately gives away your power and takes a toll on your life.

The good news for you and me is that limiting beliefs can be changed, rewired effectually, into more empowering beliefs. Scientists have been able to study neuroplasticity which is the brain's ability to learn new ways of thinking and behaving. For a long time, the science community asserted that after a particular age, the brain stops making new neural connections, but we now know that is no longer the case. Science has proven even the most deep-seated limiting beliefs can be transformed into an empowering belief system. Regardless of how old you are, with repetition and practice, your brain can be rewired. In the book *Rewire Your Brain: Think Your Way to a Better Life*, John B. Arden says, "use strengthens connections, and non-use weakens them. Old connections that are not strengthened by relationships will fade."[3] This means when you give your attention to empowering beliefs instead of limiting ones, the old belief system will slowly fade into the abyss. This creates space within your mind for a new mindset that aligns with living a healthier and happier life.

Beliefs that relate to health, fitness, nutrition, and weight loss can be some of the hardest to rewire because of the depth of our limiting beliefs. We receive messages from the media and societal expectations about what women need to look like to be happy, healthy, worthy of love, and successful. The diet culturescape is born out of preying on women's limiting beliefs through fatphobia, photoshop, and other means. It evokes emotions of shame and inadequacy. It programs limiting beliefs on all three levels: yourself, others, and the world.

I hope to show you that you don't need to buy into this mindset to live a happy and healthy life. In fact, there is a much better way to approach health and weight loss that also supports long-term well-being. The diet culturescape itself is riddled with limiting beliefs that don't support longevity nor healthy living. Nothing within the diet culturescape teaches women how to cultivate a healthy mindset. Instead, the diet culturescape exemplifies the cave, and dieters are the prisoners who are chained to the walls. Each diet, like a shadow on the wall, captures the attention of the prisoners. If you don't look at your mindset, you're likely to stay trapped, dependent on the next fad diet and your willpower. You must understand the depth of your belief systems and the power it has over your entire life because the power is yours for the taking. To change a poor eating behavior you've tried so desperately to break, we have to take three steps back to understand where it's coming from. And once you've escaped the diet culturescape cave, you will see the beauty of eating good food and loving your body.

2

THE DIETER'S MINDSET

Whether you're popular or a wallflower, you have a critic. You can't see the critic, but you can hear it. She whispers lies to you. You might be thinking, *oh yeah, that's me; I'm my worst inner critic.* The liar in your mind is not you, though. It's a belief system programmed throughout your life. Your most real self would never say *you are ugly*, or *you are fat*. Those horrible thoughts and lies are not the real you.

When we live our life without taming the liar in our head, we become slaves. The longer we allow this liar to continue speaking, the stronger the unhealthy mindset gets. The diet culturescape feeds this liar by programming many women with a dieter's mindset. The dieter's mindset is borne from the limiting belief that you are not good enough in your current body. Like a carrot on a stick, the diet culturescape dangles the image of a perfect body and happiness. And guess who's the ass?

The carrot is so close, you can have it if you try hard enough the liar says. But no matter how fast you run, you don't get any closer to the carrot. No matter how hard you work, you won't ever be able to snatch the carrot out of the air. Motivation lasts only a minute, and it's rarely there when you really need it. Yet the dieter's mindset heavily relies on it to attain unrealistic goals. Ultimately, we all get tired of chasing something that's unattainable, so we give up. Then the negative internal dialogue ensues. And here starts the cycle of restricting your diet, overeating because you restricted too much, and then feeling ashamed about failing—only to start right back at the beginning again. Alas, it was already well-known by the holder of the stick that the goal was never meant to be attainable.

The diet culturescape knows the reality of this cycle and is all about delaying happiness until your body is perfect. You cannot fully experience life until you've reached some abstract ideal weight. The diet culturescape programs women to adopt a dieter's mindset because it's the culturally and socially accepted norm. A dieter's mindset is riddled with limiting beliefs that ultimately inhibit health, vitality, and overall well-being. The limiting beliefs allow negative thoughts to run wild in your mind, which results in emotions of shame and feelings of inadequacy.

Women are taught to prioritize weight over well-being, starting as far back as childhood. It's a prison that glorifies weight loss at all costs. It's not about striving to live a vital, energetic life. It's a sad belief that happiness is conditional. It's training the mind to believe the lie "I'll be happy when I'm skinny." When we attach self-worth to external events like weight loss, money, success, or being in a relationship, that is when we rob ourselves of happiness.

A dieter's mindset develops when the diet culturescape resonates subliminal messages to your subconscious mind. The culture at large promotes thinness as the ideal. Women are led to believe that they must have a perfect figure at all costs. No cellulite, no jiggle allowed. The messages bombard your mind, like hundreds of spam emails. Over time, the external stimulus impacts your thoughts and emotions, and eventually, a belief system is planted. And this dieter's belief system makes you think things like:

> *I need to lose weight by summertime.*
> *I don't deserve to eat the foods I love.*
> *I'll always be fat.*

Carbs will make me fat.
Fat will make me fat.
I've tried everything to lose weight.
My whole family is overweight; I'm destined to be fat.
I can't eat that, or I'll gain weight.
No man will love me in this body.

These are limiting beliefs that most women with a dieter's mindset will experience a variation of at some point. These limiting beliefs are restrictive and debilitating and lead to unhealthy thought patterns, emotional reactivity, and, ultimately, self-sabotaging behaviors that contribute to unhappiness, weight gain, and diet hopping. These limiting beliefs keep you trapped in the cave or stuck on the hamster wheel, chasing after body standards that are unrealistic for the general population. Limiting beliefs are used in this space to keep women feeling ashamed about their bodies and perpetually stuck in a restrictive diet as a result. The diet culturescape is the culprit for crafting the dieter's mindset within you, which is the root cause of your unwanted eating behaviors.

The dieter's mindset is multifaceted. The main message instilled deep into your subconscious mind by the diet culturescape is that your body is not good enough. This tends to be the deepest limiting belief women experience. If you are constantly trying to alter your body, it's possible you hold this limiting belief that you are not worthy in your present-day body. This limiting belief is validated by cultural rules to keep women locked in the dieter's mindset. Over the years of healing my own mind and working with many women, I've discovered the pillars that uphold the dieter's mindset within us. A mindset that keeps us prisoners within the dieter's cave.

The first fundamental element of the dieter's mindset is self-rejection. This is the idea that you are not worthy of joy the way you currently are. Or you perpetually feel as though you're not good enough. In the diet culturescape, worth is dependent on weight and dress size. Thinness is praised, validated, and held up on a pedestal as the ideal body type—something all women should be striving to attain at all costs. Women who attempt to meet these arbitrary body standards end up experiencing more shame and rejection. Having any belief rooted in self-rejection can make it impossible to meet your own needs and truly take care of yourself. This comes from feeling unworthy of being happy and feeling good in your body.

In a study conducted in 2015, low self-esteem or experiencing self-rejection showed an increase in mental health issues like depression and anxiety[1]. To cope with these negative thoughts and emotions, women will abandon their own needs in favor of tending to the needs of others in an attempt to feel needed and recognized. Many women have been taught in the larger culturescape that they are not responsible for meeting their own needs and that, magically, by taking care of others, their needs will be met, and they will, in turn, feel happier. Women who experience self-rejection may overeat in an attempt to feel "full" inside without even realizing that they are doing it. When beliefs that encourage self-rejection are repeated for years, women are left feeling depleted, frustrated, and ashamed that they can't seem to reach the goals that diet culturescape asserts all women should be able to reach.

Another adversity of the dieter's mindset is victimhood, also known as denying self-responsibility. Many of the patients that I work with know this as "making excuses." This mindset encourages women to view themselves as a victim of life circumstances and the actions of others. It paints them as helpless to the circumstances of the larger world and leaves them reacting to external events. The limiting beliefs that underlie victimhood sound like: *I have no time to make healthy meals, I can't lose weight when my husband keeps ice cream in the house, I can't control myself around unhealthy food*. These beliefs are incredibly disempowering and strip away all your power. While you may not be able to control what other people do or what happens in the world, you always have control over your thoughts, emotions, and actions.

The dieter's mindset urges women to look outside themselves for things like validation and support for their lifestyle choices and complain instead of taking responsibility for the things they *can* control. The truth is, there are some things you can control. You can control the thoughts you choose to indulge in and the food you put into your mouth. You can control the way you view yourself and how you want to spend your time. The difference is that when you're a victim, *nothing* is in your control. You let other people and situations control your actions. You give away your autonomy and the ability to make a different choice for yourself. People or situations can't control you or get in the way of your health goals if you don't give them the key and let them drive the car. Nevertheless, life is still life, and one hundred percent of my patients experience obstacles that are out of their control.

I had a patient who constantly denied self-responsibility. She would come in week after week and report the same sort of things; she didn't have time to prepare healthy meals in advance, didn't have enough time to exercise, and blamed her husband or kids for keeping unhealthy foods in the house that she "couldn't control herself" around. By giving away her power, she was able to avoid feeling like a failure and taking responsibility for not meeting her goals, but she didn't gain anything from it. Being a victim will keep you a victim.

What my patient initially failed to see were all the places she *did* have control if she only had a different mindset. Instead of focusing on all the things she couldn't control, we started focusing on the things she did have control over. We looked at the habits and thoughts she was investing her time and energy into believing as well as the habits and thoughts she wasn't prioritizing. Just by taking ownership of her time, moderating her disempowering beliefs, and implementing small habits and routines that brought her closer to her targets, she was able to reach her goals without shame, struggle, or deprivation.

Equating food with morality is another piece of the dieter's mindset. Instead of seeing food as something to aid our health and wellness, it's viewed as a moral compass. When women have a dieter's mindset, they are obsessed with weight fluctuation as a measure and indicator of health. With the fear around weight gain so prevalent, women restrict their diets in an attempt to lose weight. These diets typically label some foods as "good" while others are being labeled as "bad." Sometimes, even entire food groups are labeled into one category or the other. Women end up fearing bad foods because they aren't allowed to eat them. This forces women to follow a highly restrictive diet that doesn't satiate them or properly fuel their bodies, and it results in them binging on the "bad" foods regardless. Women then attach the label of "bad" to themselves because they trespassed and ate a forbidden food.

The language around eating less nutritious foods is highly polarizing, making women with the diet mindset think that they are doing something wrong simply by eating. The language around "cheat foods" is also damaging. Equating food with morality leaves women feeling yucky and exasperated. They feel as though they can't eat anything and, as a result, eat everything. Assigning morality labels to foods makes women assign those labels to themselves. The belief in good and bad foods can fuel eating disorders that are prevalent in women across all races, body sizes, and ages because women are so scared to gain weight. They fear the weight gain reflects who they are and what they do and don't deserve as a result.

The fear of certain food groups altogether forces those with a dieter's mindset to try and achieve perfection. Diet culturescape instills this belief into women that they can have the perfect body as long as they eat perfect foods perfectly. The obsession with perfection is unhealthy for all of us because it leads to extreme measures in search of perfection which does not exist.

As a recovering perfectionist, I learned this lesson the hard way. Human beings are not perfect and never will be, and yet we are bombarded with photoshopped images of women that are airbrushed past the point of recognition. A 2015 study concluded that women frequently compared their body and appearance to friends, peers, and celebrities which often resulted in body image concerns and negative self-image.[2] Even when the women knew that the images were likely photoshopped, they still compared themselves to these other modified bodies. Comparison is truly the thief of joy! I know from firsthand experience.

When women don't look perfect or eat perfect, it leads to self-punishment. If you don't have a perfect day of eating, you need to go to the gym "to burn it all off," making exercise a punishment for simply eating food—something you need to do to survive. Or you overeat because you already "cheated" on your diet, so you vow to never eat another "bad" food and start restricting all "bad" foods again on Monday. The cycle of perfectionism and punishment makes it impossible for women to reach their health and wellness goals because perfection when it comes to nutrition and body size is a myth—keeping you stuck in the same behavior patterns preventing progress on improving your health.

The dieter's mindset is shaped by the external environment, and the focus is entirely outward. Outward appearance. Outward happiness. Outward expectations being met. It is also reactive to these external events. Instead of taking control and being proactive, a reactive person will let the events set life's agenda. It's emotionally responding to the external events around you. When one is reactive, one lives a life without purpose or mindfulness. Simply put, it's merely surviving. The lack of proactivity results in inhibition to choose your response.

The dieter's mindset is much like Plato's cave, given that when you're in it, you are a prisoner. But there is a better way to achieve health. You can escape the cave and experience a better way of living, and it is with a healthy mindset. The health mindset is different from the dieter's mindset because it is shaped from within. There is no culturescape you must conform to which influences your decisions. There are no disempowering beliefs that linger in your mind. And there is no link between eating and morality.

The health mindset puts you in the driver's seat. It allows you to focus on your unique body and health status. It empowers you to make the best fitness and nutrition choices for your particular life situation. The health mindset is a new perspective on well-being.

3

THE HEALTH MINDSET

As I walked onto the cardiac unit, I placed my floral clipboard under my arm so I could wash my hands. I ran my hands under the warm water with plenty of soap, scrubbing intensely. Once my hands were clean and dry, I looked at my patient list and silently repeated in my mind, *Mr. Crane. Room three, bed one. Mr. Crane, room three, bed one.* I quickly reviewed the reason I was nutritionally assessing the 94-year-old patient. Then, I walked into the room and softly uttered, "Knock, knock. Mr. Crane?" As I lifted my head from the clipboard, I saw an older man on the phone, staring at me with a pleasant smile.

"Yes, that's me," replied Mr. Crane. Then talking back into the phone, he said, "Hold on, dear, I have someone visiting me. I'll give you a call back after." He hung up the phone and looked up at me, and enthusiastically said, "That was my companion caregiver. I was just checking in on how she was doing." I was surprised by his strong, articulate voice and youthful energy. I quickly looked down at my clipboard to double-check his age because I had never seen someone in their nineties look and act so . . . young. I introduced myself and began my assessment.

With each answer Mr. Crane provided, the more curious I became to how this old man was living so vibrantly. Our conversation flowed as he told me about his life. He told me how everyone he knew had passed away, so he hired a companion (the woman on the phone). He told me about his heart condition and how the doctors told him it's because of old age. He explained how he had difficulty chewing and swallowing so he followed a blenderized diet. How could someone who experienced so many unfortunate events still be thriving? He could sense my inquisitive being, so he told me his secret: acceptance. He accepted that life is temporary. He accepted his medical diagnosis. He accepted that he couldn't eat a solid diet and expressed gratitude for his companion, who prepared soft, blended, nutritious meals for him.

"I hope you live to 100 years old so you can become a centenarian," I beamed. Mr. Crane laughed and responded with confidence that he will definitely be living past one hundred. He appreciated my encouragement and cheer.

I was so immersed in Mr. Crane's perspective on life that I forgot about time and work. I eventually realized I had to go finish my charting. It was difficult to leave this extraordinary person. As I was about to leave, I told him I was going to write a book one day and how he will be in it. He chuckled and granted permission. This stranger who I had only met an hour ago believed in me. I walked away feeling like I just struck gold. "Acceptance," I thought, smiling as I sauntered back to the dietitian's office.

Mr. Crane left a mark on me that day. He exemplifies the *health mindset*. The health mindset is not another shame-inducing diet or a cave to be trapped in. The health mindset is a step away from the restriction and perfection of a dieter's mindset in favor of seeing food as good, nourishing, and healthful. Mr. Crane didn't mind that his food was blended like baby food; he felt great knowing it was nourishing. Mr. Crane didn't act like a victim; he took things into his own hands when it came to loneliness. He knew how important social interaction is for a human's well-being, so he hired a female companion to care for him and keep him company.

Instead of preying on and exacerbating limiting beliefs, the health mindset allows you to take your own health path. Health is dynamic and nutrition is not cookie cutter. A health mindset supports choices that are healthiest for that individual based on unique wellness goals. It doesn't need to promote one ideal size, shape, or weight as the standard. The health mindset knows that a healthy body will look different for every person. By stepping into the health mindset, you leave behind the unrealistic diets and adopt a healthier way of living and being. The health mindset is not an all-or-nothing approach to dieting but allows for flexibility in your eating. In this mindset, there is no right or wrong, good or bad to control and define you—which means you can make decisions based on nourishment and, frankly, eating what tastes good! The health mindset is the beautiful, colorful, free world awaiting you outside Plato's cave.

The health mindset is about *being* a healthy person every day. Acceptance and self-compassion are at the core of the health mindset. True health isn't defined by a certain size or weight. Well-being comes from creating empowering beliefs about your body, food, and health. The health mindset encourages the creation of empowering beliefs about what is possible in this life. It's about embodying what health means to you and living that definition every day. Having a health mindset will force you to get uncomfortable in the short term to have long-term health and wellness with a focus on experiencing joy right now. Those already living with the health mindset didn't learn it overnight.

Most people get stuck in the same patterns of behaving, reacting, and thinking that cause them to repeat the same unhealthy patterns for years. But their desire for a better way to eat and live drives them forward. Just like you, they had the feeling deep down inside that something was missing, like there had to be a better way to think and feel about one's body temple and food. Most people that are ready to adopt the health mindset are desperate for freedom. Freedom from the shackles that keep them sick, sad, and hating their bodies. It all comes with fully adopting a healthy mindset on the inside to create an energized, healthful, and joyful life on the outside.

The health mindset encompasses encouraging characteristics that will help you gain control of your thoughts, emotions, and behaviors. It peels off the old layers of your identity that have existed since you were a child. It quiets the loud voice that spews lies. It strips away the power of the past and invites you to create the life you want. It does not keep you in an anxious state focusing on the past or future. As a matter of fact, *being* in the present is an important part of the health mindset.

The art of *being* is the focus on the present

moment because the past and future are mere mirages. This took me some time to fully wrap my head around. The past no longer exists, just the memory. The future also does not exist, just the imagination. *Being* is a practice of respecting, celebrating, and appreciating who you are and how your body looks *right now*. Death teaches us one main thing: your life is not promised. I don't mean to be so morbid, but at any moment, you can die. Whether you are an immoral or moral person, whether you're overweight or skinny, your body will eventually die.

You have a choice, right now, to be happy or to continue putting off your happiness for the unpromising future. I used to put off my happiness when I was in college. I believed the lie that I'll be happy once my abs were showing. I thought I would be happy once I was successful. I don't know about you, but I certainly don't want to hinge my happiness anymore on the arbitrary idea that in the future, I will be happier once I attain a better body or achieve success.

In case you didn't know this little secret to life, happiness isn't a destination to be reached. It's a state of mind that can be cultivated at any time. My happiest moments in life so far were not triggered by any external event. Sure, I was happy when we bought our first house. I was happy when I graduated college and got my first dietitian job. But there's a bliss I've experienced far greater than the relative happiness and it doesn't stem from external events. Stop waiting to live your life until the weekend, until you're thin, or until you're happy with the way you look in a bathing suit. Life will not stop to wait for you, and it's a gift to allow yourself to *be* in this moment and experience all it has to offer.

There was a patient that I worked with who struggled with her weight for years. As we began working together to address her limiting beliefs, her behaviors started changing. She started picking foods that nourished her body and movement that made her joyful. It didn't take long for her to lose some weight and achieve the better health she desired. The week she was no longer deemed prediabetic, I was thrilled, but she didn't seem as happy. When she came back for her appointment, I asked her if there were any noticeable mindset shifts from the week before. She told me she had been upset last week because she noticed people were treating her differently now that she was thinner (this *can* develop into a limiting belief). People held doors open for her, were more friendly to her, and even her husband was being nicer to her. It began to bother her, so she decided to speak to her husband about it. She then told me that she had it *all wrong*. Her husband told her people weren't treating her better because she was thinner; they were treating her better because she was treating the world differently. She continued, telling me she was in fact friendlier to strangers, she was smiling more, started singing in the shower again, and taking care of herself in a way she never had before. After talking to her husband, she realized that it was her new health mindset all along. By rewriting her mindset, she changed her perspective on life, and was able to achieve happiness and health like never before.

While the dieter's mindset promotes victimhood, the health mindset offers responsibility. Taking responsibility for the things in your life can be hard and intimidating at first because you remove other people from the equation. When you blame other people or the world for your problems, you give away all your power. You are merely left to react to the world, letting other people control your environment, behavior, and emotions. Taking responsibility for your life is both exhilarating and frightening. There is no longer a husband to point to and blame or children that can be your scapegoat; your success in anything starts and ends with you.

With the heaviness that comes from accepting responsibility for everything that happens in your life, there is also the freedom that accompanies it.

THE HEALTH MINDSET

The freedom that you get to choose your thoughts, emotions, and actions. You are in control of all those things that build your life and your identity. Taking your health into your own hands doesn't mean that you're responsible for working out every day or eating your vegetables at every meal, but it means that you take control over the things you have control over. The health mindset is the serenity prayer:

> *God grant me the serenity*
> ***To accept the things I***
> ***cannot change;***
> ***Courage to change the***
> ***things I can;***
> ***And wisdom to know the***
> ***difference.***
> *Living one day at a time;*
> *Enjoying one moment at a time;*
> *Accepting hardships as the pathway*
> *to peace;*
> *Taking, as He did, this sinful world*
> *As it is, not as I would have it;*
> *Trusting that He will make things*
> *right*
> *If I surrender to His Will;*
> ***So that I may be***

> ***reasonably happy in
> this life
> And supremely happy
> with Him***
> *Forever and ever in the next.*
> *Amen.*

You have the power to shape your perspective and align yourself with doing things that will bring you closer to your dreams. And just like Mr. Crane, you will eventually develop innate wisdom to know when you must accept something you cannot change. No one knows your life as much as you do. You might be struggling with an undiagnosed medical condition, or you might have a child on the spectrum. You might have an increasing reliance on a numbing substance, such as alcohol, tobacco, or marijuana. The health mindset encourages you to stay centered, conscious of the present moment, and committed to remaining open.

The words 'acceptance' and 'respect' are listed as synonyms in the dictionary, but each has a nuance that separates the two. Regardless, both radical acceptance and self-respect are qualities of a health mindset. Radical acceptance in this mindset is accepting your body just the way she is. It means that you're not obsessing over trying to look like a

Victoria's Secret model or pining after other bodies as you scroll through Instagram. Radically accepting your body is when you allow it to exist without picking it apart. It's knowing that your best and healthiest body *won't* look like anyone else's body, and it doesn't mean that your body is weird, wrong, or meant to be changed.

Radical acceptance comes from a place of self-compassion. Self-compassion is when you are kind to yourself and accept your humanness. You are not the only one struggling with negative body image or poor eating behaviors. Being mean and hard on yourself hasn't gotten you results in the past, and it won't get you the results you're looking for in the future. You can't heal a body you hate. Giving yourself some grace when you make a mistake cultivates self-acceptance. It ends the war you have been upholding for years and allows space for inner peace.

Self-respect is different in that it doesn't ask for us to simply acknowledge all bodies are valid but also that we deserve to treat ourselves with honor and dignity. Self-respect takes radical acceptance just one step further because it asks you to treat your body now the same way you would treat your body if it were "perfect" or "the ideal." Right now, no matter your age or size, or weight, you deserve to be treated with honor and dignity by others, and you deserve to treat yourself that way too. The more you learn to honor and respect yourself, the kinder you talk to yourself and the better you feel. When you feel better, you do things that make you feel good too.

Respecting yourself means fueling your body with tasty nutritious foods and honoring your body with movement. A great place to start showing your body more respect is through practicing gratitude. I could write an entire book on gratitude alone because it has proven to be a powerful, albeit underutilized tool that helps the most entrenched prisoner release themselves from the cave. Results from a 2018 study about body image found young people practicing body-focused gratitude had less internalized weight bias than the controlled group in both males and females.[1] Simply practicing gratitude as it relates to your body can help alleviate some dieter's mindset beliefs. Your body is one of a kind, and it deserves to be loved, honored, and cared for—and you are the only one who can do those things for yourself. We will dive deeper into gratitude and other practices in a later chapter.

The health mindset recognizes there is no "one-size-fits-all" approach to modern-day eating. The dieter's mindset of restriction and cookie-cutter diets falls on one end of the spectrum. However, there is another school of thought that says, "Eff all diets!" This is the other extreme that doesn't take health into account at all when it comes to eating, which can lead to physical problems. Both dietary dogmas interrupt personalized nutrition. The health mindset exists somewhere in between these two, like a grey area. In fact, the health mindset prioritizes grey thinking over black and white thinking. This means that there is no restriction on the foods you're permitted to eat, but there is still an emphasis on eating healthfully. It means not only paying attention to and being aware of the foods you consume but also how they make you feel. You can be at your desired weight *and* eat pizza. You can have curves *and* be metabolically healthy. You can eat veggies *and* ice cream. The health mindset prioritizes grey thinking because it mirrors reality which is *entirely* grey.

Things are not as simple as good and bad or right and wrong; many times, these ideas are layered and nuanced, with much of the categories bleeding into one another. Grey thinking allows us to move away from binaries like "processed foods are bad" into more realistic thinking like processed foods if eaten in excess are not good for our health, but they do allow for preservation, convenience, and are often fortified with nutrients. The latter allows us to understand more of the full picture and the reality of the situation as opposed to simply lumping it into one category. When you live in the grey area, it is much easier to have respect, compassion, and acceptance for yourself and your body if you're courageous enough to try.

Courage is not something that is typically touched upon when it comes to eating, but it's an essential point of discussion in the health mindset conversation. There is so much fear surrounding food indoctrinated by the diet culturescape. This fear of eating takes over many women's lives. The process of feeding themselves becomes confusing, hard, overwhelming, and exhausting because they are so scared to do the wrong thing.

When fear saturates your body, it triggers a stress response. When you feel fear, your brain releases chemicals that put you into a fight, flight, or freeze mode. When your fear response has been triggered, your brain can't tell whether you're getting ready to outrun a tiger or considering a second cookie for dessert. Your body responds to any stressed state in the same way—shutting down the digestive system, raising blood sugar, dilating pupils—getting you ready to run for your life.

Chronic stress can induce headaches, high blood pressure, shortness of breath, all of which can make it harder to choose nutritious food.[2] Stress can compound over years if left unmanaged and can result in body inflammation. When you can release stress and fear, you are no longer being controlled by your animalistic fight-or-flight responses. This release and physiologic transition will improve digestion and allow for a clearer mind so you may make better food choices that are aligned with your health.

Courageous eating also means that you eat for joy and celebration as much as you do for nourishment. Fearless eating is eating the salad you prepared for lunch at work *and* the cookie your coworker baked for you. It's eating a balanced, nutritious breakfast *and* Christmas dinner with your family. Eating is not meant to induce fear. Both nutrient-dense foods, as well as treats, are meant to be savored with joy!

Eating without fear requires learning to trust yourself. It means tuning into that wise voice inside of you that already knows what you need when you need it. Some might say that it's a voice, others call it a gut feeling, but most know it as intuition. Intuition is the ability to understand something immediately, without the need for conscious reasoning. Some call this sensation innate wisdom, while others allude to a spiritual connection to a higher power. Regarding health, it is biological feedback, information from the body to the brain about what it needs and wants to operate at its best.

Your intuition wants your body to thrive and function optimally. Have you ever felt the itch to move your body? Or started craving a juicy piece of steak? I know after a long vacation where I'm eating out for most meals, I find myself craving vegetables, particularly roasted broccoli. These are examples of your intuition, communicating what your body needs. Most of us have become so numb to the sensations in our bodies because we spent years denying and ignoring them.

Learning to listen and respect your body's cues is a powerful characteristic of the health mindset. If you've been neglecting your intuition, you will need to relearn the process of quieting the other, much louder voice, the liar. Intuition doesn't tend to have a loud voice. It requires checking in daily on how your body and mind feel. Intuition is a muscle; the more you listen, the stronger it gets. Also, have some faith in yourself throughout the process. Yes, you may struggle and have setbacks in the beginning, but it's important to trust that your body knows what it needs.

The health mindset is an incredible upgrade from the dieter's mindset because you are no longer reacting to the world around you and allowing the beliefs of other people to dictate how you view yourself and how you live your life. The health mindset is deliberate; it's a conscious choice that reflects who you really are instead of what the diet culturescape commands you to be. You don't need to look like an influencer to be happy. You don't need to restrict yourself to be healthy. The health mindset encourages you to be the best and healthiest version of yourself every single day. It allows you to make the rules about health based on your unique body, needs, and preferences because it acknowledges that health is not one-size-fits-all. It considers you as a whole human that was not put on this planet just to be thin. You are a person who has a purpose, and you are meant to create a meaningful life. And to do this, health is your biggest asset. When you feel well, you live well.

The health mindset encourages you to eat nutritious food because it makes you feel good and gives you energy, but also promotes balance so you can live your life unrestricted. Foods like cake, cookies, and ice cream won't ever disappear, and that's why the focus is not on completely eradicating them. Instead, the focus is on learning how you can uphold your health with balance and allowance.

Health is dynamic as it is continually changing with the progression of your life. Like Mr. Crane, you will get older, and your definition of health will change. You no longer need to eat by means of hype or fad, but personally, through self-respect and intuition. Well-being is the result of accepting the things you cannot change about your body with compassion and love. During puberty, child-bearing years, and menopause, the body will change. It is normal and it is beautiful.

The health mindset is a strong foundation on which you build your healthiest and happiest life. So, when things get a bit bumpy, and they will, not everything will crumble. A loved one may pass away. A relationship might end. You could lose your job. It is up to us to strengthen what's on the inside to withstand the pressure from the outside. Life is dynamic and ever-changing, and we too must be dynamic with our mindset and health.

4

AWARENESS

It's easy to notice the differences in mindset when I spell it all out for you here, but it's another thing entirely to put it into practice. Ditching the dieter's mindset isn't easy because it is pervasive and exists everywhere. It exists at the office among co-workers who grapple for hours over whether they should eat a slice of pizza. It exists when you go out to dinner with friends who talk about how little they ate all day. And it exists in the wall of your very own mind when you put on jeans that are too tight. If it was easy to overcome the diet culturescape, I think we would have way more people thriving in their bodies. The truth is while many of these concepts are simple, they are not easy.

The key to changing your unwanted behaviors is *awareness*. Remember, it was awareness that truly freed the prisoner from the limiting beliefs of the cave. It is through your awareness of your current belief system that allows you to transform your mentality from a dieter's mindset to a health mindset. Awareness is one thing I coach all of my patients on because for you to be able to change anything at all, you must be conscious of it. To recode a negative limiting belief, you need to identify what the behavior/emotion/thought/belief is and, ultimately, understand what triggers it.

Most of the behaviors we perform throughout the day are largely unconscious and automatic. Once our brain learns how to do new things, it will automate doing them to save energy. When we bring awareness to these often-bypassed areas of our lives, we create space to change them. You move from simply reacting to your external environment to being able to thoughtfully respond in a way that aligns with a happier and healthier life.

It can be uncomfortable when you start becoming more aware of behaviors, emotions, and thoughts because most of them tend to be negative, but you're not to blame. Humans have what is called a negativity bias, otherwise known as a propensity for negative thinking as opposed to positive thinking.[1] Most scientists accredit this phenomenon to a survival need; that we need to be on the lookout for tigers hiding in bushes so we can get a head start on outrunning them. Our negativity bias is what helped to keep us safe in the past. The key is to gently observe yourself going about your life and notice what comes up. Use awareness without judgment. There is no room for shame or guilt here, and it's important to be gentle with yourself in the process.

There are four keys of awareness you'll need to unlock and free yourself from the corners of your internal prison. Using the first key, you will understand your current eating behaviors. The second key releases stored emotions. The third key allows thoughts to enter your awareness. And the fourth key frees you from limiting beliefs. Utilizing the awareness keys, you will create space for a new belief to be written.

The first awareness key is to discover your typical eating behaviors. Remember, there is no judgment here, so it's important to be honest with yourself. You aren't dissecting your eating habits to berate or belittle yourself. You are trying to become aware for the betterment of your health. Take a deep breath and remember that you are merely observing, and you are not labeling the things you observe. If anything, get curious about your eating habits and try to view it as information you're collecting. It helps to keep a journal or write notes on your phone to track findings and patterns in behaviors.

Behaviors are what you *do* in response to a *stimulus*. Do you eat in response to feeling stressed, overwhelmed, or sad? Are you mindlessly eating while watching Netflix or scrolling on your phone? Grazing all day? Binging large amounts of food all at once? Finishing every scrap on your plate, licking your plate clean? Observe your behavior during your next meal and write down the things you notice. Instead of logging your food or counting calories, your job is to take notes on your behaviors, emotions, and thoughts while eating.

Next, use the second awareness key to discover stored emotions. Observing emotions can be difficult because sometimes feeling an emotion is highly uncomfortable. Emotions are energy moving through the body and can cause all different sensations from a racing heart to a sinking stomach. It's important to remember that emotions are just energy, and it's safe to acknowledge and feel them. Emotions need to be felt, processed, and released. And remember, you are not your emotions—let them pass.

A short disclaimer here. If any of these emotions become too difficult for you to feel, please, please, please reach out to a professional. Yes, I'm saying to get yourself a therapist. It's a wonderful tool to support your mindset transformation journey.

Emotions are a common trigger for unhealthy eating behaviors. If you've jotted down a couple of eating patterns, go one step deeper into understanding what emotion drives each particular eating behavior. Do you feel stressed from work before you overeat dinner? Do you feel bored before you mindlessly eat while watching TV? Continue to keep notes in a journal or phone. Write down what emotion you're feeling. If you're not sure, check in with your body. Increasing awareness of your emotions associated with eating will help you better understand why you have trouble changing an eating behavior. For example, if you eat ice cream whenever you're feeling stressed, that might explain why cutting out sugar a month before a big work deadline didn't work.

Notice how you feel during your meal. Do you feel shameful, out of control, impatient, calm, or happy? Observe if your mood changes at all throughout the meal or stays the same.

Finally, once your meal is over, write down how you feel again. Are you feeling overwhelmed, insecure, angry, peaceful, or relaxed? How about self-rejection or self-sabotage? When you are able to bring awareness to your emotions, you are able to utilize non-food-related coping skills to manage those emotions and bring yourself into a happier, more joyful state when munching for a happier eating experience.

The next area to investigate is your thoughts. The third awareness key is used to bring thoughts into the conscious spotlight. Your goal here is to find what thoughts are impacting your emotions. If you discovered a pattern of feelings of guilt when you ate a certain food, what thoughts are causing that emotion to arise? Common negative thoughts around body image and food are:

> *I'm fat.*
> *I hate how I look in the mirror.*
> *I might as well finish off the cookies*
>   *since I'm already a failure.*
> *Carbs are bad.*
> *[insert literally any food] is bad.*

Many different thoughts might come up from the diet culturescape that have been swirling around your cranium *undetected*. Just know that you're not alone. The diet culturescape heavily influences women's thinking, and if left in their hands, it continues to mold mindsets every day.

A systematic review published by Nutrition &

Dietetics in 2019 affirmed that women ages 18–30 know that social media impacts their body image and food choices, but they still want to conform for peer validation.[2] The diet culturescape isn't going away. It's up to you to weed out the disempowering thoughts and practice deliberate thinking. The more disempowering thoughts you can bring into awareness, the easier they are to get control over. And those disempowering thoughts will lead you to the root cause of your unwanted behaviors, your limiting beliefs.

Finally, we will take all of the information we've collected about your behaviors, your emotions, and your thoughts to unveil your limiting beliefs. This fourth key is the most important because this is the root of all your thoughts, emotions, and behaviors. Most of the time, limiting beliefs come from childhood and teenage years. Remember, these are the years where most of our beliefs form. It's at this impressionable time that we learn the rules of life from friends and family, and often those beliefs don't empower us or serve our well-being.

One common limiting belief is women thinking that they will be happy when they've lost some weight or toned a body part. This belief all but prohibits you from being happy right now. Not only are you not allowing yourself to be happy, but the truth is that nothing external will ever be able to make you happy. Joy comes from within and requires one to find the happy things purposely every day. Happiness comes from who you are and how you spend your time. It will never come from size two jeans.

Another limiting belief that women have is that no one will date you or love you if you're fat. This belief truly breaks my heart because it limits a loving partner from entering your life because of your weight insecurity. Many overweight women are happy with their bodies and have partners who love them, just like there are skinny women who have partners who despise them. Weight should not stop a person from loving you.

If you have trouble pinpointing your limiting beliefs, reflect on the things you heard your parents say a lot in relation to food, health, and body size. Did your mom call herself fat? Did you grow up poor with little food available? Looking back at your childhood experiences can be helpful in accessing a deeper sense of self-knowledge, which is incredibly powerful when trying to make a change.

Examining where these beliefs originated can be useful as you work on getting to the root of your limiting beliefs. How and when did the beliefs start? Identifying who was involved and what happened can be helpful to expose the roots of these limiting beliefs.

Often, we let things that happened in the past mean something about us, and we hold onto it as part of our identity for most of our lives without ever asking; is this true for me? The stories of your past shape your present and future. The more you get to know yourself on deeper levels, the more you can look at the darker parts and process them as a rational adult, the more clearly you will see yourself. And one day, you will realize you have been living in a cave, starved of self-compassion, respect, and genuine happiness. Some of the moments where our limiting beliefs began don't seem like big, important moments in retrospect. It could be something as small as your best friend skipping lunch because she says she doesn't want to get fat, or it could be something much larger that jumps out at you.

One patient I worked with went through this whole process with me, and at the end, she told me about the moment she began thinking about her body in a negative way. It was an evening when she was watching her mom get ready to go out to dinner. Her mom looked at herself with disgust in the mirror and made a comment about being overweight. My patient estimated she was about eight years old at the time. She had always thought her mom was beautiful and perfect. It wasn't until she noticed the way her mom spoke about being overweight that made my patient start to become self-conscious of her own body. She grew up with a fear of food because she didn't want to be overweight. Her insecurity and limiting beliefs launched her into the dieter's mindset, where she struggled with her body image and relationship with food for years.

It wasn't until she uncovered this deep-rooted insecurity from this interaction with her mother that she began to understand the reasons she was struggling with food. She realized she believed if she was overweight, her mother wouldn't love her, or worse, would think she was disgusting. That moment, where her mom wasn't even directing the comment or attention to my patient, shaped her relationship with food and body for most of her life.

I had another patient who came to see me to help her heal her gut, and she wanted to have more energy. She really struggled with her eating. She either ate extraordinarily little or ate a super large meal all at once. After taking some time to identify her behaviors, emotions, and thoughts, she noticed a pattern. She would restrict her food very severely all week long, and then she would binge on the weekends. She noticed that before she binged, she felt ashamed or deemed herself a failure. She knew going into the meal that she was going to overeat because she had deprived her body of nourishment all week long. She would feel great while eating, but as soon as she was done, the self-rejection would come back into play. She had thoughts like: *carbs will make me fat, I am fat, I don't deserve to eat.* Her major limiting belief was fat people don't deserve to eat and feel full. Restricting put her on an unhealthy eating cycle.

After working with her for a few weeks, she came to see me with a breakthrough. She remembered as a kid, her parents often told her she was fat and wasn't allowed to have seconds at dinner. Often, she also wasn't allowed dessert. Her brother, on the other hand, wasn't fat, so he could eat whatever he wanted. She was able to see how her behaviors, emotions, and thoughts came into play to feed into her limiting belief; that fat people don't deserve to eat. Once she identified all of this, she was able to go into meals with awareness and a plan for overcoming those disempowering beliefs and all that flow from them.

Uncovering these deep-seated negative beliefs helps us to heal them. What remains hidden deep in our subconscious minds needs to be brought up to the surface so we can understand it and change it into something else. Sometimes, examining these memories can be painful, but once you begin to understand and get to know yourself, it will get easier, and you will begin to transform. Some of the limiting beliefs you have now are the same beliefs you've had since you were a child. It's time to update your belief system to match where you are in your life right now and to help you get where you want to go.

You are in control over your mind. Awareness results in the expansion and power over your mind. You no longer need to be a victim to the same limiting beliefs; find yourself stuck in the same patterns. As you begin to exit the cave, it will feel as though a light has been brought to the dark corners of your psyche. The thoughts that were once cemented into your mind as an opposition begin to dissolve. With those thoughts gone, it's so much easier to address the daily habits that keep you stuck repeating the same unhealthy patterns. You are able to choose new habits to replace the old ones—habits that align with the healthier and happier life that you are trying to live, but it's a process. The journey is not linear, meaning there will be good days and low days, but you will find that over time the bad days will decrease in number until it's mostly great days. Hang in there, keep your awareness on, and don't give up.

5

REWIRING YOUR BELIEFS

I HAVE GONE TO GREAT LENGTHS TO REWIRE MY OWN limiting beliefs, from reading every self-help book to practicing meditation to utilizing sensory deprivation tanks. And through all of the alternative therapies I've used and all the books I've read, there is one common message I kept on receiving; *I am not my thoughts or my emotions.* After years of struggling with anxiety that would roll around my mind unchecked, I felt the waves of peace wash over me as I stopped identifying with my thoughts.

Thoughts and emotions are something that all humans experience, but they are not something we should be victims to. The thoughts you have and the emotions you feel all come down to your belief system, which can be altered and changed. Learning this, knowing this, set me free. Thoughts and emotions are phenomena that occur within me, but they are not me. You have the ability to choose your thoughts and even choose your emotions. Therefore, you do not need to be a victim or slave to your mind. *You* are the one in charge, and you can decide whether you want to stay trapped in the cave or whether you are ready to see the light of a different kind.

Once you identify your personal limiting beliefs and start proving that some aren't necessarily the truth, it's time to focus on unlearning them or replacing them with something much more empowering. Without uprooting the old beliefs, we have no room to plant new ones. Unlearning old beliefs is hard because you have spent so much of your life unconsciously validating them. Instead of uprooting a dandelion, you are trying to uproot a 25-year-old oak tree, and that kind of uprooting shakes the foundations of who you are at your core.

Rewiring your mind and creating new habits takes time. As Dr. Caroline Leaf says, "It takes a minimum of 63 days to change an automated habit- when it comes to the mind, there really are no quick fixes, and most people give up on day 4, so be patient!"[1] You can choose new habits to replace the old ones, practices that align with the healthier and happier life you are trying to live, but it's a process that starts with becoming aware of your belief systems.

You've probably discovered a couple of limiting belief systems by now (and if you haven't found any, get yourself back to the previous chapter—this is accountability, girl). Observe the thoughts that surface from the depths of your limiting beliefs. What thoughts arise when you get ready for work, on your commute home, or when you make dinner? The goal of this mindfulness practice is to become aware of the thoughts that do not serve you. It might be helpful to keep a running list in a journal as you're working on simply observing what these thoughts are. You do not need to change anything just yet. You might realize most of your negative thoughts stemming from limiting beliefs have been swimming around your head constantly! It is through gaining awareness of your thoughts that you may discover where they are coming from.

The other day, I was driving to work and noticed a fly zooming around inside my car. It was slightly distracting as I am not a big fan of bugs, so I rolled down my windows, and within a couple of minutes, the fly escaped the confines of my vehicle. Like a fly trapped in a car, thoughts are trapped in your mind. We need to open the window so distracting thoughts have an opportunity to get out.

Opening the window to our minds can be a bit tricky, though. The best method of release is writing your thoughts down. Putting pen to paper is a powerful exercise to clean your mind of unnecessary thoughts. Freeing thoughts will create space in your mind for your new healthy belief system. Writing is putting your brain on paper. You can cleanse your busy mind by doing a brain drain writing exercise in the morning, or you can keep a note on your phone as you discover repetitive thoughts that do not serve your well-being.

Utilizing all four awareness keys (awareness of behaviors, emotions, thoughts, and belief system), you can remove the implantation of a limiting belief system. As you move through each day, ask yourself some serious questions. Are these beliefs *really* the truth? Does it align with your values? Are the thoughts empowering you to feel joyous, confident, and fulfilled? If they aren't, ask yourself *why*.

If you haven't already started writing down some of your discoveries, I give you permission to go to Target and buy the cutest lined journal you can find. Or grab a piece of copy paper or sticky note and a pen. Just start writing whatever comes to mind for five minutes. It can even be: *This woman is crazy. I effing hate journaling. This is a waste of my time.* This clearance exercise provides room for new thoughts. Practicing this daily will speed up the rewiring process of the brain.

It's not enough to just stop thinking about the old thoughts. This fearful reaction pushes unwanted thoughts further into your shadow or subconscious mind, the deeper part of the iceberg. They don't disappear down there and will continue to pop up in your mind over and over again when triggered. You must welcome the thoughts that do not serve you and gently release them. Then you can begin to give your attention to the more empowering beliefs and ideas.

Once you have created space in your mind after releasing negative thoughts, you have room to instill a new thought process. You can use positive affirmations to take up room in the space you just created to combat repetitive negative thinking. Positive affirmations are mantras and phrases that are empowering and align with your values. Affirmations are powerful because they help us create a new, empowered identity and typically start with the phrase "I am." Anything that comes after that short and simple phrase is powerful because this is where you recreate your identity. Some of my favorite affirmations for rewiring limiting diet culturescape beliefs are:

I am loved, and I am worthy of love from others.
I approve of me.

I am safe in my beautiful body.
I am wonderful just the way I am.
I create my own sense of security.
I am happy, and I am courageous.
I am able to meet my needs with ease and joy.
I am proud of myself.
I love myself more each day.
I am the caretaker of this wonderous body temple.
I am beautiful inside and out.
I am good enough.

An affirmation should not feel forced. Instead, it should resonate with you and generate feelings of love and acceptance. Some people find it helpful to write down their affirmations every day, but I recommend saying your affirmations aloud. Hearing affirmations in your own voice tells both your conscious and subconscious mind to pay attention and listen. The more you repeat these affirmations, the more likely they are to stick (remember back to the previous chapter about rewiring; your brain will strengthen the connections that you give attention to). Write your affirmations on a post-it note and stick them on your mirror, set your affirmations as the background of your phone, or even set the alarm to go off twice a day, prompting you to repeat your affirmations out loud. Make this a practice that reenergizes you to continue down the path to cultivating the health mindset.

There was a patient I worked with for months who struggled to rewire her thinking. We were working on increasing her overall fiber intake to support her weight loss and health. I tend to save the last five minutes of our sessions to review any potential obstacles that may get in the way of success. It was right around the 4th of July, and she mentioned a family barbeque she had to attend over the upcoming long weekend. As we talked about the impending holiday, she expressed worry about the event because there was never any healthy food available on these occasions. She didn't want to upset her family members by not eating the foods they cooked. I listened intently and asked her what from her past was making her feel that way. She explained that as a kid, her family always made her feel guilty or bad if she didn't eat the food they prepared for her. As a child, she didn't have the autonomy or confidence to advocate for herself and her food choices. So she had to eat the things her family made, even when it was unhealthy, and she didn't enjoy it. She thought that's just the way it was.

Together, we uncovered a limiting belief: *I will make my family upset if I don't eat the food they prepare, even if it's unhealthy or not what I would prefer to eat.* Now, as an adult, she realized she didn't have to subscribe to that belief. During the remainder of our chat, she came up with a new, more empowering perspective that restored her power by giving her the gift of choice. Her new belief was: *I respect my health every day and can choose to bring food that aligns with my health goals, and I enjoy eating.* She also decided to pick a mantra to repeat when she noticed old thoughts surfacing. She chose: *I am the caretaker of this amazing body.* This switch in her mindset gave her the power to ditch victimhood and to make the best choices for herself. Becoming aware and changing the language in this belief prepared her to go to her family event confidently.

The following month during our follow-up session, I asked her how the barbeque went. She enthusiastically reported that it went great! She prepared two dishes she loved, an Asian salad and roasted brussels sprouts. She said that some of her family members gave her a hard time for not eating all the dishes they prepared. However, she was able to tell them kindly she would like to stick to the foods that made her feel her best and politely declined the things she didn't want to eat.

Did some people initially get a little upset? Sure, they did. Especially since their pattern of behavior was to use guilt and shame to coerce my patient into making unhealthful choices for herself. But because she rewrote the belief system, she didn't sway in her thoughts, emotions, or behaviors. She told me that her old limiting beliefs popped up occasionally, the fear that she wouldn't be loved if she didn't eat the food her family had prepared, but she allowed them to pass through. She anticipated the negative thoughts, and she had a positive affirmation ready to keep her aligned. Making one small change to her belief system helped my patient gain control over her life, even if it was just for a day. The feelings of freedom, joy, and self-respect that came with this little win propelled her to do more work on her limiting beliefs. Now, she doesn't have her old limiting beliefs visiting her as often and consciously builds the foundation of her health.

There is a superpower that dwells within each of us: gratitude. Being thankful is another way to support the rewiring of your limiting belief systems. I have firsthand experienced the magic of gratitude, and it has become a non-negotiable part of my morning routine. When we focus on the things we don't have, we are more likely to feel sad and deficient. Distorted thinking is a major cause of suffering. Gratitude is the practice of consciously expressing thanks and feeling appreciative for what you have in your life now. It includes being grateful for your amazing body! Gratitude is well known to improve overall well-being by increasing feelings of happiness in those who practice it on a regular basis. It can have the same effects when implemented to focus on being thankful for things that relate to self-image and nutrition. One study found that teens who expressed gratitude reported healthier eating behavior over time.[2] This means simply by being thankful and expressing gratitude related to body image and nutrition, people improved their eating habits.

The other day on my lunch break, I drove over to my favorite smoothie shop to order an açaí bowl. As I sat there enjoying one of my favorite meals, a feeling of gratitude overcame me. I was grateful to be able to eat the meal without pain. You see, the majority of my patients have digestive issues, so eating and pain are, unfortunately, closely related in these patient's minds. You can probably understand how pain might impact one's eating behaviors. I observe this every workday, so how can I not be grateful when I don't have pain after eating? It's these little acts of gratitude that rewire your brain and increase true happiness. And honestly, my açaí bowl tasted ten times better with the side of appreciation.

Spend five minutes every day, or, heck, right now, to shift your mindset to one that is positive, thankful, and joyful by writing down what you're grateful for. Here's my health gratitude list to exemplify how simple this practice is:

> *I'm thankful for my body and everything it does to keep me alive.*
> *I'm grateful that I can go for a walk around the block.*
> *I'm thankful to have access to the nutritious food I get to eat.*
> *I'm grateful to be alive without pain and present in this moment.*
> *I'm thankful for my morning black coffee and clean water.*
> *I'm grateful that I have healthy choices available to me.*

One of my favorite gratitude practices is my "thank you" walk. It's an intuitively paced walk around my neighborhood. With each step I take, I say *thank you* in my mind. Then, after about ten thank you steps, I expand the gratitude to the different aspects of my health. I am thankful for my leg muscles. I am thankful I can walk without pain. I am thankful for my breath and the fresh air. I am thankful for my digestive system. I am thankful for my brain and vision. And if I run out of things to be grateful for or my mind wanders, I return my focus back to being thankful for each step I am able to take. *Thank you. Thank you. Thank you.*

Having gratitude for your body doesn't mean you don't want to improve or that you're ignoring very real health complications. It's just the practice of training your brain to see all you *do* have instead of what you lack. You won't get anywhere if you're committed to seeing everything in a negative light. A negative mindset will never lead you to positive results. Choosing to find the good right where you are is what keeps life fulfilling, even when it gets tough. Training your brain to be appreciative is more motivating than berating yourself ever will be.

Another patient I helped was highly motivated to lose weight and improve her health. She was super dedicated and told me that she would do whatever it took to begin repairing her health and rid herself of the excess body weight she felt she was carrying. She was unhappy with her appearance, and her superficial motivations were primarily aesthetic. She wanted to be more confident, happier, and thinner. After talking about nutrition basics, she was still hesitant to eat carbs and healthy fats in moderation. She would grossly undereat, and on the days she did eat more, her diet was made mainly up of microwavable Lean Cuisines, fat-free foods, and other heavily processed foods. Her dieter's mindset and limiting beliefs kept her fearful of eating nutritious foods and stuck in the same eating patterns. She relied on the rules of the diet culturescape, which kept her in the same cycle. After working to bring awareness to her eating behaviors, emotions associated with eating, and thoughts about food and her body, the indoctrination became clear to her. She started the process of rewriting her limiting beliefs, but she still complained of "feeling fat" and was frustrated that massive shifts weren't immediately happening.

That's when we introduced gratitude. Adding a new habit into a morning routine can be challenging, so we decided to pair her gratitude list with her morning coffee. She bought herself a pretty journal and vowed to give it a try until our next session. When she returned for her follow-up two weeks later, she was thrilled to tell me that she felt better than ever. Almost every morning, she made her list of three things she was grateful for while she took the first few sips of her coffee. Not only had she stuck with her gratitude journaling, but she was really feeling more thankful for her body every day. She explained how she began appreciating her body. She started making healthier choices for herself—choices that were more in line with a healthy mindset. She had a newfound appreciation for the nutritious food she was eating. She transformed her perspective from "I have to" to the powerful "I get to" attitude. When she did enjoy less nutritious foods, she took the time to enjoy and appreciate them and didn't feel out of control around her eating. Gratitude created new brain connections within her mind and changed her lack mindset into an abundance mindset.

Along with journaling, affirmations, and gratitude, meditation is a powerful tool for rewiring limiting beliefs and has been getting major attention from the science and psychology communities in recent years. There are different ways you can go about meditation. You can try to clear your mind; you can practice mindfulness; you can listen to a guided meditation; you can focus on your breathing. Like dieting, there is no cookie-cutter way to meditate.

The goal of meditation, like journaling, is to declutter the mind and create space. However, sitting in silence and completely clearing your mind is more challenging than it sounds. Initially, it feels as though your brain doesn't ever fully turn "off," moving a mile a minute. It's when we close our eyes and relax our bodies that the brain sees an opportunity to bombard us with thoughts. Anyone with anxiety or insomnia knows this feeling well as they lay their head on the pillow at night but cannot fall asleep because of their active minds.

Meditation teaches practitioners to observe passing thoughts and then bringing back awareness to the present moment. Meditation has been an effective tool in increasing positive emotions and self-compassion.[3] Meditation sometimes feels blissful, joyful, and unique, while other times, it feels like it's a waste of time and nothing is happening. Those that claim they can't meditate are the ones that need it most. Just know that even if it doesn't *feel* like anything is happening on the surface, your brain changes with each meditation session you partake in. Mindfulness meditation, also known as focused reflection, has been well studied and shows promising brain changes after eight weeks of practice.

If you are a beginner meditator, let me walk you through a typical meditation session. It's best to set a timer for five or ten minutes. This will allow you to forget about the dimension of time, which rules our reality. Once your timer is set, sit or lay comfortably, preferably in a place where you don't usually sleep (this will help you stay awake and get your brain into the best frequency for mediating). If you are a beginner, minimizing distractions, such as pets, family members, and phone notifications will support your practice. Once you have created the ideal setting, bring awareness to your body, and focus on your breath. You can count if you'd like. Five counts for your inhale, five counts for your exhale, experiencing the top and bottom of your breath for a couple of seconds. Notice any sounds you hear in the room or outside. Are they close or far away? Bring awareness to how your body is feeling. Notice the space your body is taking up in the room. Feel the weight of your body pressing into the chair or the floor beneath you. Feel those body parts grow heavier, and, starting down at your feet, observe your body. Can you relax your feet more? How about your calves and thighs? Continue scanning your body, letting go of tension, allowing the ground beneath to support you.

Once your body is somewhat relaxed, bring your attention and awareness to your thoughts. What is going through your mind right now? As you let thoughts enter your mind, picture them as a butterfly. The butterfly floats down and lands at the front of your mind. Observe it for a moment, and then allow the thought to release and send the butterfly flying on its way out of your mind. Continue to do this until your timer buzzes.

Each time you meditate, try to add another minute to your timer. At first, you might feel like you're checking an email box with 10,000 emails that are all bombarding you for your attention, and that is normal. Allow the thoughts to come and go, and it will get easier—I promise! As you improve mindfulness meditation, you can expand your practice to visualization, connect with your intuition, and ask more profound questions.

Who are you really . . . at your core? The great philosophers tried to answer this question of "Who am I?" Meditation reveals to us that we *are* the awareness. Your thoughts and emotions will come and go, yet you remain. Every seven years, you essentially become a new body because old cells have been replaced by new cells. Your body ages, but *you* don't. You are so much more than just a body or mind; you are a soul/spirit/being brought here to dance and laugh and sing and love. You're here to create, learn, and experience life. To line-dance your heart out at your favorite country club, run around with your kids kicking the soccer ball in the backyard, and enjoy exquisite foods while on a tropical vacation. You are a human *being* equipped with the tools needed to cultivate well-being: a state of health and happiness.

Take your rightful seat on the throne of awareness. This life is your life, and you deserve to live it fully without excessive thoughts about food and poor body image taking up room in your waking mind. Like the thought leaders, uncover who you are beneath the layers of societal conditioning. And then remind yourself who the heck you are every day. You are the editor of your life, and you decide what thoughts and emotions deserve your energy and which do not.

As you move through different phases of your life, you will likely uncover new limiting beliefs. The more you learn how to identify limiting beliefs, the more you will begin to notice there really is no end to them. I realized this truth after years of therapy. You heal one area of your life only to discover more limiting beliefs in another area to address. This is a constant process of learning more about yourself as you evolve through life. For example, entering a new relationship, starting a new career, getting married, or having a baby will likely bring up limiting beliefs to the surface. As they come up, rewire them using the keys of awareness and tools of intentionality, and you will continue to level up.

As you align yourself with the health mindset, it's important to focus on acceptance and respect as well as grey thinking, courage, and intuition. Creating a new, healthy mindset and reality requires action. The uncomfortable yet necessary steps are why many people choose to remain locked up in a cave, allowing their limiting beliefs to dictate their life stories. It's those that identify with their past who have a hard time moving forward. Get out of your own way by releasing attachment to old identities. Take a breath and appreciate how far you have come. As you cultivate a health mindset, your body will undoubtedly follow.

6

REWRITE YOUR DEFINITION OF HEALTH

IT'S A WARM, SUNNY AFTERNOON ON THE FIRST DAY OF fall in the year 2117. I'm sitting on my granddaughter's couch dressed in my favorite yellow dress and comfortable white shoes. As each family member arrives, they rush over to hug me. The little ones comment on my soft wrinkly skin and how shiny my grey hair looks. The sound of my favorite music fills the air. As I sit in my old body temple, feelings of joy and love pass through me. It's my 123rd birthday.

I recognize an upbeat song playing in the background. A song I used to sing at the top of my lungs as a young woman. One of my great-granddaughters embraces my hands as I slowly rise to my feet. I start to sway, moving my body to the music and taking total delight in the moment. My family joins in dancing around me, singing along to Taylor Swift:

> *Everything will be alright if*
> *we just keep dancing like we're*
> *twenty-two; twenty-twooo ooo*
> *ooo ooo*

In my mind, this vision is my *why* for living a healthy lifestyle now. I have this desire to feel alive every day. Like, *really* alive. I want every day to be filled with lots of laughing, dancing, and playing. Not just now, but also on my 123rd birthday and every day in between. I don't want to spend time pining after someone else's unattainable body or picture-perfect life. I want joy and love in my life right now under the current circumstances, whether good or bad, and every day that follows. I want to be able to dance with utmost joy when I break the world record for the longest human lifespan! The oldest human to have ever lived (with full documented proof) is Jeanne Louise Calment, who lived to 122 years old and 164 days—a true triumph. I want to be thriving when I'm that age, not merely surviving. There is no time like the present to start embodying the joy and vitality I crave, and the same goes for you.

You might not care about living a long life. Maybe you're one of those people that wants to drop dead at 65 years old, so you never have to face the reality of pooping your pants or forgetting your child's name. All that is fine and valid. The point is that the state of everyone's current health is different, and we all have individual goals. The diet mindset restricts the conversation about health to weight alone rather than redefining health for each unique person. The health mindset encourages women to think about health in ways outside of weight alone. Health comprises of many different moving parts, and physical health is only one category. Weight is merely a subcategory of that.

I want you to know it's okay if you want to tone your arms or tighten your booty. If sculpting your body is something that's going to boost your confidence, girl go for it. But don't allow aesthetics to take primary importance in your decision to living a healthy life. It will end in disappointment because your beautiful female body is going to change over the years and decades. During puberty, your body changes. During your twenties, your hips get bigger. During your fertility years, body fat is wonderfully important when you're growing a baby human inside of you. Then, after you've created life, your body changes again. And so on. And once you're in your seventies, body fat becomes protective yet again as appetite tends to cease.

The dictionary definition of health is "the state of being free from illness or injury." The diet culturescape has also defined health. Healthy, as defined by the diet culturescape, is slender, tight, with smooth skin. The diet culturescape ties health directly to what your body looks like, but health encompasses more than that. As the bland dictionary definition states, health is being free of disease. Health encompasses mental health, physical health, spiritual health, and emotional well-being, among other things.

Your definition of health should encompass these different facets in ways that are important to you. What health looks like for your specific body, mind, and soul will differ from my vision. Health looks different for everybody, and you can't tell whether or not someone is healthy based on just weight alone. I've seen plenty of patients who have a hot body but are internally sick. And I've seen my fair share of overweight patients in their seventies, in good health. Health differs from body to body. And you might have your own idea of health, depending on if you have any medical conditions or have a family history of diseases. Since you are the creator of your life and know yourself best, define what healthy looks like for you. My patients have described health in a multitude of ways, for example:

> *Health is having energy when my grandkids come over.*
> *Health is preventing Alzheimer's my mom suffered with.*
> *Health is reversing my diabetes.*
> *Healthy is feeling alive and well throughout my day.*
> *Healthy is living pain-free.*

Before we get into writing *your* own definition of health, let's go over some housekeeping. No matter what your health goals are, there are some non-negotiable components of health I can't let you ignore. We haven't gotten this far in nutrition science to proclaim that solely eating Snicker Bars will optimize your health and support longevity if you *really* believe it will. And while I'm sure you can cultivate a mindset that tricks your body into remaining healthy without taking care of it, science is still science. And as a dietitian, I want to give you the framework of healthy living so you can thrive in that beautiful body temple of yours!

The four pillars of health are nutrition, movement, rest, and spirit, all of which are built on the foundation of the health mindset. What you eat, how you move, how much you rest, and how connected you are to your true self all equate to your health. We will discuss eating well at length in the next chapter, but the other pillars should help guide you as you write your definition of health.

The human body was made to move. So even if you cringe at the thought of exercise or groan begrudgingly, movement plays a significant role in our overall health, including mental well-being. A systematic review published in the *Journal of Happiness Studies* found all the studies reported positive associations between physical movement and happiness; even as little as ten minutes a day or one day of exercise per week can increase happiness levels.[1]

Despite the positive effects of movement, people have a love-hate relationship with exercise. I'm here to tell you that movement doesn't need to be the most painful part of your day. Exercise is not punishment because you ate too many calories. People typically equate movement with grueling kinds of exercise; lifting heavy weights, running for miles, sweating, grunting, and struggling to catch your breath. If that's the type of movement you enjoy, by all means, have at it! But there is more than just one kind of movement to support health. Movement can be going for a power walk around the block or a peaceful stride on the beach. Movement can mean dancing in your kitchen as you prepare dinner for the family or vacuuming and tidying up your home. Movement can include playing with your dog baby, gardening, playing a sport like tennis, or simply stretching your body every hour. The key with movement is finding something you enjoy doing and fitting a little bit of it into your week for a happier and healthier life.

A common limiting belief about exercise I've encountered with patients is: *I exercise to burn off excess calories*. We can use the healthy mindset framework to see that this belief tells us there is only one reason to exercise, but we all know that isn't true. There are dozens of reasons to exercise, ranging from heart health to wanting to be able to outrun zombies in the event of an apocalypse. With intent, we can change that limiting belief into something more empowering like: *I exercise because it makes me feel good and improves my mood*. This new belief isn't punishing or shameful. Instead, it reminds you how alive you feel after moving your body.

In the example above about exercise, the limiting belief equated exercise with punishment. In whose right mind are pain and punishment a joyful thing (excluding those into *Fifty Shades of Grey*)? This belief leads those to think: *This will be hard, I won't enjoy it, exercise is pain.* That kind of thinking makes us feel bad when we don't do anything wrong. With a new empowering belief, we will find thoughts such as: *What movement can I implement today that will help me feel my best? What exercise can I choose today that will improve my mood?* These thoughts not only make us look forward to movement, but it's also freeing knowing that you can choose any kind of exercise you want. It doesn't have to be a backbreaking workout to reach your goals.

While movement is necessary for health and longevity, so is rest. American culture seems to be allergic to rest. My female patients have the worst relationship with rest and don't truly understand how rest impacts overall health. We believe that our worth is tied to *doing* instead of *being*. We must do all the things: take care of others, have a successful career, keep our home tidy and aesthetic. While it's important to have a clean space and to give attention to these areas of our lives, we also need unapologetic time to rest. To feel our best and most vibrant selves, we need time for our mind, body, and soul to properly recover from the stress we constantly put ourselves under.

True rest is when you give yourself permission to

take a day off from producing (this is a hard one for us workaholics). It's allowing yourself to enjoy playtime with the kids even when there is laundry to fold or dishes to clean. This type of rest allows you to simply exist and enjoy the gifts of life around you without constantly needing to jump to the next thing. Rest can do wonders for your body and spirit.

The pillar of rest also prioritizes sleep. If you're the kind of person who thinks that five hours of sleep is enough to function, you may be right, it's *just* enough to survive. But is that kind of rest enough for a rejuvenated life that increases your sense of well-being? No. Anything less than six hours of sleep is considered inadequate. Sleep is necessary to reset your body so you can thrive the next day. Stop accepting "just enough to get by" in all areas of your life, including rest. Prioritize sleep and observe how you blossom into the happiest and healthiest version of yourself.

In these periods of rest, it's also important to take care of your spirit, the fourth pillar of health. If you're reading this and wondering what in the heck it means to take care of your spirit, you're not alone. I know it's a woo-woo topic, but I've found that those who don't actively take care of this area of their health, feel less excited and energized about life.

Other terms to describe spirit include soul, being, self, inner child, awareness, consciousness, etc.

Investing in your spirit speaks to who you are outside of your career and relationships. Spirituality does not concern the material and physical world. To promote spiritual health, reconnect with your inner being. Your true self is not your loud ego and does not communicate with words. It speaks through intuition using feeling and energy. Your inner being is not your thoughts, emotions, nor is she your body. She is the one who comes from and is connected to the highest source of love. It's this faith in a higher power that reveals the purpose for your life.

If you feel completely disconnected from this true self of yours, don't worry. The good news is, you don't have to go out looking for her because she's already right here within you. Ask yourself what makes you light up or feel mighty. Think about the activities that boost your confidence and strengthens the connection to your intuition. What excites you about life? What makes you feel aligned with the infinite being you are? Your answers are the things that are important to your spirit. To nourish your inner being is to fill up a cup. Spirituality is a lifelong journey that parallels and supports the path to health and happiness.

Your happiest and healthiest self does not do the bare minimum in any aspect of life, including self-care. All areas of your personhood deserve love, attention, and energy for you to bloom into the greatest version of yourself. Carving out time in your busy schedule to do things that make you feel energized and joyful is the key to a sustainably happy and healthy life. Invest in your hobbies, try new things that excite you, explore your interests, fill up your own cup so that you have the energy and motivation to fulfill your purpose.

Understanding the pillars of health outlined here are all designed to catapult you forward to living your best life. It's not about restricting yourself, doing exercises that you hate, trying to get by on minimum rest, or denying yourself true joy and freedom. It's about using the knowledge to expand our definition of health.

Keeping the pillars of health in mind, you can effectively rewrite your definition of health. Throughout the process of rewiring your mind, it can help to take note of your values. Most of us go through life without ever taking inventory of the traits and principles that are most important to us. Pay attention to whether you are living in alignment with your values. If you value adventure, how often do you experience adventure? If you value intellect, what's the last book you read? You may have a stark realization that you're not acting in alignment with your values at all. What would your life look like if you acted in line with your standards? How can you embody your values every day?

A couple of things I value are freedom and authenticity. I value freedom of choice and freedom to experience cool and exciting things life has to offer. However, when I had my old diet mindset of restriction, there was misalignment. How can one encounter freedom when one also must restrict? A restriction mindset does not align with a freedom mindset and both drive separate behaviors. I also value authenticity, yet when I was obsessed with my body image, there I was taking a gym selfie with my body perfectly positioned.

If you need a little help ascertaining your values, here is a list of common values:

*adventure, authenticity, autonomy,
balance, beauty, compassion,
community, contribution,
creativity, fairness, faith,
friendships, fun, growth,
happiness, honesty, humor, inner*

harmony, justice, kindness, leadership, loyalty, optimism, peace, respect, security, self-respect, service, spirituality, stability, success, trustworthiness, wealth, wisdom

Circle, highlight, write it a hundred times. Do what you need, girl to keep it at the forefront of your mind.

The pillars of health and values you hold near and dear to your heart work together to create the roadmap to living a more joyful and vitalized life. I don't want to see any more women attempting to squeeze into the mold created by the diet culturescape when there is a whole world of health that awaits them outside of that narrow-minded way of thinking.

Now, it's time for the fun part: imagine your happiest and healthiest self. Forget the timelines and travel to the future where this beautiful self exists. There are no rules to the imagination! Allow your values to fuel this vision of your healthiest self. What does she look like? How does she spend her time? How does she feel every day? What sort of choices does she make about her health? Does she take medications? What boundaries does she have? How does she feel about and talk to her body? What makes her feel her best every day? What does she do to take care of herself? What is her sleep like? Picture all the details of your highest self. Then, write down everything about this version of you. Dream big here, and don't skimp on the details. Again, this is your life, your dream! Why not create a life that is as amazing, healthy, and joyful as humanly possible? Health is available to you, and this exercise serves as the destination on the map to well-being.

After you've visualized what health looks like on you, it's *finally* time to grab a pen and write down *your* definition of health. What does "health" really mean to you? Go on, write it down now. Is health being able to walk without heavy breathing? Is health feeling energized all day long? There is no wrong answer. Here are some examples to spark inspiration if needed:

- *Health is feeling radiant and beautiful inside and out.*
- *Health is experiencing a clear mind throughout the day.*
- *Health is eating my favorite foods joyfully without guilt.*
- *Health is choosing nutritious foods to promote a long, energetic life.*

- *Health is moving my body in a way that feels good.*
- *Health is giving myself permission to rest so I may give my best to the world.*
- *Health is keeping up with my grandchildren.*
- *Health is accepting my natural body size with kindness and compassion.*

Read your definition every day, once in the morning and again before you go to bed at night. Repeat it like a mantra whenever you encounter old limiting beliefs. Allow this definition of health to take root in your mind and spread the word to all the cells in your body. Your new definition of health and your rewritten beliefs should empower you.

As you expand your consciousness with your new definition and ditch the baggage of your old limiting beliefs, you'll notice other changes start to happen. New thoughts will trickle in flowing from your new belief system. The more you invest in embodying your empowering beliefs, the more encouraging your thoughts become. Your thoughts are like little streams flowing from the pool of consciousness. Where attention goes, energy flows. As your thoughts run off this larger pool of belief, positive emotions will arise.

Limiting beliefs will continue to rear their ugly head sometimes, like when you're under stress from work, experiencing hardship, or trying to implement new things. As long as you don't pour all of your energy into giving those limiting beliefs power, you will stay on track with your thoughts, emotions, and actions. Stay committed to your health journey; remember it is not linear. When you give yourself permission to take responsibility for your health, you can better handle the curveballs life throws at you. With every challenge, there is also a multitude of solutions. It's your perspective that enables you to catch the opportunity for growth or miss it. The health mindset increases your openness, and you might just start to notice the little opportunities you would have otherwise missed.

Identities get in the way of us living out our vision. In the Bible, there's a story of a man who had been sick for thirty-eight years, waiting by this healing pool. Jesus asked the lame man a simple question that we all need to ask ourselves. *Do you want to get well?* The man offered excuses as to why he couldn't, dodging the question. And so do we. Why do we identify so heavily with our hardships? Why do we get so comfortable with our illnesses that it becomes a source of safety? At the beginning of my career, I thought the answer to Jesus' question was a no-brainer: O*f course, my patient wants to get well.* So, I gave my all to teach every single patient how to eat well, pouring my energy into each sick person. The unfortunate truth is not every patient I see wants to get better. Some people are more comfortable with their discomfort. And this was a hard pill for me to swallow.

Ask yourself: *Do I want to get well?* If your answer is yes, then mean it. Commit to your *yes*. Check in with yourself to see if you identify with anything that might get in the way of your healing. Do you identify with being the "fat girl?" Do you identify with being sick all the time or disabled? Do you identify with a diet tribe like keto or vegan? These identities will unconsciously find obstacles on your path to well-being.

When you make the single decision to get well, in body and mind, you become proactive instead of reactive. This is emotional intelligence, and it boils back down to awareness. Becoming aware of your body's natural cues is an integral part of controlling your emotional response. When you are unconscious of your emotions, you snap at people unknowingly. You take your stress out on the people you love. You might even emotionally sabotage yourself. Having emotional intelligence means that you practice awareness of your emotions. As a result, you have control over how you express them. This practice takes time, but as you align with your definition of health and increase mindfulness, your emotions will be easier to manage. This may look like going for a walk when you're feeling frustrated instead of emotionally eating. It may look like going to sleep on time instead of forcing yourself to work past the point of burnout. These self-serving thoughts offer time and space to process your emotions in new, healthy ways that are in alignment with your values and beliefs that keep you living out your healthiest and happiest life.

The more you begin to believe in yourself and your unlimited potential to have the happy and healthy life of your dreams, the more likely you will be to act on it. If you believe well-being is not possible for you, you will never take the action that supports your health. Simply believing that something is possible for you means you are halfway to achieving it.

Embracing your new healthy emotional state will spur new behaviors. When you successfully make a behavior change that aligns with your definition of health, it's important to celebrate! Implementing new behaviors is tough, and whenever you take a step—big or small—toward accomplishing your health goals, it is worth celebrating. Giving yourself a pat on the back for your success and showing yourself adoration makes it more likely that you will engage in those behaviors again in the future. Think about a little kid in your life. Suppose you praise a child for doing a positive thing and making a good choice. They will continue to engage in positive behavior. Within your subconscious mind resides your inner child who needs praise for displaying good behaviors. Make sure you're giving yourself credit often so that you stay motivated to make choices that support your empowered mindset.

Your beliefs control everything; your thoughts, emotions, and behaviors which is why they are the key in releasing the limiting diet mindset and wholly embodying the health mindset. Keep your new, empowering definition somewhere you can see it every day in order to keep the energy flowing toward your self-empowerment. In the beginning, you will notice that rehearsing these beliefs takes conscious effort and energy. You may even think it's stupid or a waste of time. But in order to encode your new definition of health into your belief system, you will need to remind yourself often to ensure your mind is rewiring to serve your health goals and dreams. The more you can rehearse this definition of health, the more you will take action. The more action you take, the more the health mindset will become second nature to you. This means that even when your old conditioning gets triggered, your new belief will be readily available to counter it and keep you on track. This practice takes commitment and continued awareness, but the payoff is a lifetime of freedom and joy around health and nutrition.

This awareness will help you align yourself with health every day. My favorite activity for aligning with the healthiest version of myself is to do mundane activities as if I were *her*. I walk like her. I go pee like her. I brush my teeth like her. I put on my workout shoes like her. I'm going to do these activities anyways, so why not *be* her while I do them. When you take small steps towards living your happiest and healthiest life, you will find you eventually end up making significant changes. Giant steps towards better health aren't huge at all. They are the culmination of a lot of little steps that you have mastered. Envisioning an alignment with your healthiest self will allow you to feel what it's like to have the body of your dreams.

Sometimes I like to imagine my happiest and healthiest self walking on the shore of my favorite beach. She is joyful, abundant, and worthy simply by existing. My highest self effortlessly makes choices that support her health and happiness every day without resistance. She finds gratitude and joy all around her; the sand under her feet, the sun warming her shoulders, the tickle of ocean spray on her arms and legs. My higher self is the part of me that is limitless and infinite. The part of me that knows anything she wants can be hers. She is compassionate, humble, patient, gentle, and wise. She is not afraid to set boundaries around her energy, beliefs, or time because she knows how valuable she is. She understands that everything in life starts and ends with the relationship that she has with herself. She makes that relationship a priority every day. Then, I visualize my current self walking up to her, and as she feels my presence, she turns around gently, smiling. She is happy to see me because it reminds her of how far she has come. But to me, the current self, she is everything I want to be. She is my highest self, and she is within me.

Your definition of health will be entirely your own. The thoughts you must think, the emotional changes you must make, and your actions need to support what *you* believe are the proper steps for you to take in your health journey. You have a higher self that lives inside of you, too. A higher self already knows what is best for you and what will make you feel the most joyful and abundant. The aspiration is to step into that version of yourself whenever you can. Call upon your higher self to show you the way. Doctors and dietitians will always be there to help guide you in living your healthiest life if you need them, but you are the one living inside your body. You are the one with the internal wisdom and knowledge that it takes to embody and live your healthiest, happiest life. Believe in yourself and know you are worth it. The freedom you crave is outside the cave, waiting for you to step into the light.

7

EATING WELL

I USED TO HATE VEGETABLES. I THOUGHT IT WAS hilariously ironic since I was studying to become a dietitian. I forced myself to eat them, though, because of their nutritional value. This old me feels so foreign now because these days, I find delight in eating nutritious foods, including vegetables. I love adding as many different vegetables as possible to my meals. Physiologically, my body changed as I started eating healthier foods. I naturally craved less sugar and more nutrient-dense foods. This is the reality of what happens when you change your eating behaviors with the intention of lovingly care for your body temple.

Eating well is not one-size-fits-all. Both the extremely health conscious and the anti-diet activist take eating to two different ends of the health spectrum. One side tends to equate health with eating a perfect diet. This is the typical diet culture that contains toxic tribalism. *You can't eat any sugar; it's terrible for you. Drinking celery juice will cure your illnesses. Avoid all animal products.* Then there's the other side, which doesn't equate health with body size at all. They eliminate weight and discipline entirely from the health equation. They also exemplify toxic trialism. If you aren't weight-inclusive, you are against them. If you believe a patient should lose weight for health (i.e., fatty liver, type two diabetes, metabolic syndrome), you are canceled. The anti-diet culture makes eating nutritious foods seem like a bad thing. And you need to have treats daily because *that's* freedom! They act as if you're sacrificing pleasure and joy if you're trying to eat more healthful foods like spinach, walnuts, and beans.

We tend to complicate eating because we rely on information from the loudest person on the highest platform. But there is no one perfect recommendation for nutrition. How food interacts in your unique body is dependent on genetic and lifestyle factors. Your mind also plays a big part as well. If you believe a food item is going to hurt you, your body will respond to that belief. Therefore, developing a good relationship with food is essential. The best way to nourish your own body is by turning inward. You don't need to explain your choices to everyone. You are your own project.

My philosophy for eating well is somewhere in between these tribal extremes, in the grey area. I've seen sick and healthy people of all shapes and sizes. The number on the scale is irrelevant to an extent, especially if it psychologically disturbs your well-being. However, weight loss can be included in your definition of health. To feel good in one's body is entirely dependent on *your* description and values. You don't have to fall under either side of indoctrination. You can be somewhere in the middle, implementing practices from both.

Eating well is one of my four pillars of health, and it is the one pillar that is massively overcomplicated in just about every possible way. The amount of misinformation is overwhelming and can make even experienced nutritionists scratch their heads. That's why I felt called to have a whole chapter dedicated to the principle of eating well. To provide clarity and direction on eating well for health. I mean, it is a nutrition book, right? At this point, I hope you've ditched perfectionism and procrastination (that is, waiting until Monday to 'start') as the health mindset doesn't support these shame-inducing behaviors.

There are two relationships to keep in mind as

you continue to encode the health mindset through eating well. Indeed, all contentment in life comes down to the relationship you have with the things around you. The first is your relationship with your body. What is your current relationship with your body? How did this relationship start, and how has it changed over the years? The second is your relationship with food. Do you experience any negative emotions about food? What does your eating behavior tell you about this relationship with food? Aside from ongoing nutrition studies that tell us what foods make up a health-promoting diet, your relationship with those foods can make or break it.

I'm not sure why people gravitate towards meal plans when eating is not rigid like that. What if you don't feel like eating tilapia tonight? Or what if you had an intense workout this morning and need something with a little more *oomph*. Meal plans don't encourage learning; instead, they shout *copy me*! And if you can't replicate, it leads to feelings of inadequacy, which, as we know now, is not helping us on our health journey. Your DNA is unique, and it will respond to food differently than the next chick.

Eating well is not eating perfectly. Eating well is so much more than eating "healthy foods." Eating well involves cultivating awareness, allowing you to pause and listen to your body. Eating well encourages you to be conscious of what you are eating but not in an extreme or self-deprecating manner. Eating well aligns with your definition of health.

You intuitively know what foods nourish your body. If someone were to ask you which foods are most nourishing, I guarantee you would be able to list a bunch of healthful foods. In case you *do* need a dietitian's answer on which foods are the most beneficial, let's think back to a time when the dieter's mindset didn't exist. If we rewind back to 300+ years ago before diet culture and fad diets became prominent, humans ate whole foods that grew naturally from the Earth. Foods like vegetables, fruits, nuts, seeds, and beans. Humans also ate high-quality proteins from animals that lived happy lives, grazing on green grass in a sunny field or sea animals swimming in unpolluted waters. Carbohydrates, protein, and fat were all acceptable and encouraged. There wasn't an industry to highly process our food, nor was food readily available like it is today.

One of my favorite moments working as a dietitian is when a patient experiences what it's like to feel *physically* good after adding nutritious foods to their diet. They forget about the number on the scale or the dress size, and they describe this feeling of well-being. *I just feel better. I have more energy throughout my day. It's like a fog has lifted.* The moment a patient experiences the physical benefits of eating nutritious foods is the moment of no return. I feel confident from that minute on that they will continue to add healthful foods to their diet. And if/when they stray, they will feel the difference.

So, as we intuitively know which foods make us feel energetic and well, there is another component to support eating well: intuitive and mindful eating. Intuitive eating is checking in with what *your* body needs. It's honoring hunger and respecting fullness cues. It's discovering the pleasure and satisfaction that one can find in the eating experience. It recognizes that food will not solve emotional problems. And finally, intuitive eating is honoring your health by eating foods that make you feel physically good.

Mindful eating is the ultimate tool for enjoying the eating experience. Most people eat the same way they go through life, unconsciously. We eat distracted by social media, phone games, or TV shows. We eat quickly running the kids to soccer practice, mindlessly shoveling whatever is convenient in our mouths without a second thought. We eat on our commute because there is no boundary between work and health. When we eat mindlessly, we often overeat or undereat. We eat without actually experiencing any part of our meal, and we disregard how our food makes us feel. This leads to eating well past the point of fullness or eating while feeling utterly out of control. Eating is an act of nourishment and enjoyment, but you cannot begin to tell if what you're eating nourishes you or whether you enjoy your food if you don't stop to bring your awareness to it.

Mindful eating is the practice of being present during your meals. When you eat mindfully, you allow your body to work synergistically with your mind to experience the food you eat. There is no need for your mind to focus on the past or the future. Mindful eating asks you to be attentive and attuned to your body and your meal in front of you.

As you practice mindful eating, it helps to remove any distractions (especially screens!). Before eating, take five slow, deep breaths. Feel the air come in through your nose and out through your mouth. It can be helpful to count your breaths in and out to help bring your awareness to your body in the present moment. Mindful eating provides a moment to pause and assess intuitively how you are feeling and if your behaviors align with your highest self. Mindful eating calls on using all your senses to experience the food you're eating.

Using all your five senses while you eat keeps you grounded in the present moment. It creates a profound experience with your meals and keeps you in touch with the sensations happening in your body.

Staying in tune with your body's wants and needs will guide you to what your body truly needs.

Using your sight, observe what your food looks like. Any chef will tell you we eat with our eyes first. Is your plate colorful? Is there steam rising from the hot dish in front of you? Does the food you're about to eat *look* appetizing?

Before you take a bite, use your sense of smell. What spices or scents can you notice in your food?

With your sense of touch, notice the texture and feel of your food, even if you're using a fork or knife. Is your food crispy or soft? Is it hard? Wet? Are you maybe using your hands and can feel a rough taco shell or a soft pita?

Next, using your hearing, notice the sounds of your food. Is it sizzling on your plate? Does it crunch when you bite into it? What does it sound like when you chew? Do you hear slurping?

Finally, as you eat your food, pay attention to how it tastes. Does it taste spicy or savory? Is anything on your plate bitter or sweet? How about salty? Is every bite the same, or are some bites different than others? Does your food taste delicious or bland? Using all these senses, really focus on enjoying the entire eating experience from start to finish.

Being mindful of all five senses slows you down and asks you not to rush through eating like it's a chore. Eating is an experience just as much as a concert or vacation is an experience. Most of the time, we focus on piling the next bite on our fork instead of enjoying the current one. We're focused on our next activity rather than the activity we're currently engaged in. It might seem maddening for my impatient readers who rush through their meals, but this practice is worth it. At the start, it might be hard to eat your meal mindfully but take it in steps or stages. At first, mindfully eating will look like taking one bite of your food at a time and chewing it well. Whether it's a chicken sandwich or vegetable stir-fry, each bite captures your awareness. As you start flexing your mindfulness muscle, slow your practice down even more. It might look like savoring the sweet flavors of the brownie your daughter baked. Eventually, you might give gratitude to every human that made this bite possible (the farmers, the delivery people, the cook).

The health mindset is not about eating perfectly but encourages you to find moderation and balance in your relationship with food. While the dieter's mindset encourages black and white thinking—to either eat only "health" foods, some of which are highly processed and devoid of nutrients—without allowing any room for you to eat the foods you enjoy. It can be frightening for some to eat without restriction, but this is where the grey-thinking terms moderation and balance come into play.

Black and white thinking can lead to mental health issues down the line that further impact your limiting beliefs and make it harder for you to adopt a health mindset. Embracing a health mindset means living in the grey area, getting comfortable listening to your body, getting in tune with your hunger cues, and trusting them. The more you learn to fuel your body with whole foods and allow yourself to enjoy other less healthful foods without guilt, the better you will start to feel. Leave the binary thinking in the dieter's cave.

Black and white thinking exists because it helps humans feel safe and secure. There are only two options, and one is right while the other is wrong. This type of binary thinking can help children make choices for themselves at a young age, but the comfort we get from this type of thinking as adults hinder us. When we are focused on right or wrong, all or nothing, we miss the endless amount of possibilities in the middle ground. Alternatives that still create order and boundaries but in a much healthier way. By only allowing room for extremes, you cover up the spectrum that most people live their life.

When you find black and white thinking coming up for you, such as labeling food "good" or "bad", during this process of eating well, it's important to challenge those limits to find the truth for you. One thing that can be helpful to support grey thinking is being conscious of the words you use. Ditch the limiting language like:

Always
Never
Nothing
Everything
Bad/Horrible

Using language that is extreme undoubtedly trains your mind to see things in an immoderate way. Investigate your black and white thoughts by asking yourself if that thought is really *always* true. Be honest. Let's take the example "sugar is *always* bad". The truth is, sugar is an enjoyable part of any birthday, thus it is not *always bad*. Or what about putting ketchup, which has sugar, on your omelet with mushrooms, onions, spinach, and bell peppers? In this context, ketchup is *good* by adding flavor to your highly nutritious meal.

Most of the time, you can find plenty of evidence that your black-and-white thinking is not the truth, and acknowledging the grey area helps you to see the other possibilities better. Looking for solutions to a challenge you are facing likely exists in a grey area. Let go of the rigid way of thinking that keeps you stuck in the black and white mindset. The more you allow yourself permission to live with grey-colored glasses, the more accessible the eating well principles become.

Eating well looks different for every person, but a common thread unites the health mindset. The term "well" can be defined as "in a good or satisfactory way." The healthiest people I've ever met are people who still eat dessert occasionally or enjoy a glass of wine after dinner. They eat with their health in mind but still allow room in their life for the things they enjoy. The difference between those who enjoy their food and those who restrict and don't enjoy their food is their mindset.

As a dietitian, I recommend my patients follow the 80/20 rule when it comes to food. This guideline means striving to eat healthful, whole foods, like vegetables, fruits, legumes, nuts, seeds, and high-quality animal protein 80% of the time and allowing less healthy foods to make up the remaining 20%. Trust me, eating nutritious foods 80% of the time is enough. And enjoying a less nutritious meal occasionally will not diminish your health. It's okay to have a side of ranch with your carrots and broccoli. It's okay to add some whipped cream to your berries.

You can have a piece of bread with your vegetable soup. The 80/20 rule creates room for all the forbidden food like pasta and bread, burgers and fries, ice cream, and cookies. It's about allowance, so we don't trigger restriction or deprivation. Here is a friendly reminder to avoid taking this rule back to the dieter's cave of extreme rigidity, beating yourself up if, on a particular day, 60% of your diet comprised processed foods. I give you permission to find the 80/20 balance over time.

Eating well is both a form of self-respect and self-love. Build the relationship with your amazing body that digests your food and transforms it into energy. Your body is a beautiful machine that works in ways you may never be able to fathom fully. Speak kindly about your body and the food that provides energy. Give your food and your body pep talks before you sit down to eat. Loving yourself means appreciating your body for all it is and all it does for you. It also means knowing what foods upset your belly and what foods make you feel satiated, and which leave you wanting more. The more you cultivate a healthy relationship with food and body, the easier it is to eat well because you're not endlessly chasing some extreme that is not in alignment with who you are. It's about allowing yourself to eat less nutritious foods when you crave them without mindlessly over-indulging.

When you embody these beliefs, you will find that you want to treat your body like the temple it is. The more intimately you know your body, the better you can give it what it needs so you can feel your best. You may find that you want to nourish it with food that tastes good. Eating nutritious foods demonstrates care and is ultimately an act of love for your body. When you feel good and nourished on the inside, you reflect those things on the outside too.

8

TRUST YOUR BODY TEMPLE

IT'S MIDDAY IN EARLY DECEMBER AS I GENTLY PACE IN the hospital room. A quirky, energetic woman walks in, and from my sister's previous descriptions, I know it's the doctor. "Are you ready, Michelle?" she asks my sister, who is sitting up in the hospital bed. The doctor positions me at my sister's right leg, the nurse at her left, and my brother-in-law, Ed, at the head of the bed. Looking at a monitor, the doctor says, "Okay, push." The nurse begins counting to five at the start of each push. My sister does her best with the first round of pushes. In between contractions, the doctor does a little coaching. By the third round, I join in with the nurse, counting *one two three four five*.

Everyone in the room is encouraging, "You're doing great, Michelle!" After a few rounds of pushing, I can start to see the top of my niece's head.

My cheerleading voice ceases to be clear as I choke up with awe. I feel my eyes swell as I watch her enter the world. I witness her first millisecond of life outside her cozy womb. The nurses quickly clean her up and gently place her on my sister's chest. Ed and I gather around my sister, staring at this new life, taking her first breaths. Within the first hour, she gets familiar with the boob area and drinks her first source of nutrients. Interestingly, my new little family member knows exactly what to do. She suckles, pees, poops, cries, and sleeps. This little baby's body thrives naturally.

That afternoon was one of the coolest days of my life. It added to the wonderment I have for the human body. How miraculous the female body is to create life and then birth it! How astounding is it that a woman can create the perfect concoction of nutrients? And, of course, how marvelous it is for a little baby to know instinctively it must obtain nutritious milk from its mother.

We go through life disregarding what a miracle our bodies are. We spend plenty of time looking at our thighs and stomach and face, but what about the inside? What about the hurricane of chemical reactions occurring in each cell that keep you alive? And the fact that your heart beats one hundred thousand times in one day. Or what about your digestive system that digests your food and converts it to energy? Anyone that's taken an anatomy and physiology, or biochemistry class can appreciate the extensive list of functions that keeps a human body alive. Your body is an intelligent creation that runs better than even the best man-made machines.

We tend to overlook what it's like to inhabit our one and only body. The sensation of breath flowing in and out of your lungs as you hike up a mountain. The sense of heat radiating off your cheeks when you're about to kiss someone for the first time. The feeling of your heart beating as you stand to give a speech at your best friend's wedding.

We spend so much time in our minds and not nearly enough in our bodies. This imbalance leads us to ignore the messages our body sends. The mind tries to control the body instead of trusting it. The liar in your mind demands you to change your body for the sake of pleasing the ego (AKA the mask we put on for the world). However, if we can make it a habit to connect with our body, trusting it for what it truly is, *both* the mind and body can flourish.

The truth is your body is a vessel that holds something special: your soul, spirit, *being*. It is the only body you get in this lifetime. The fact that you, yes you, are alive today is a miracle. The fact that we were born on Earth where we can live comfortably, breathe the air, and that our most precious resource —water—rains down from the sky are all an absolute miracle. Humans have been on this planet for thousands of years, and our bodies hold far more wisdom than we tend to give credit. We believe that we can logic our way out of health or physical ailments when we need to trust that our body knows the way *before* our logical mind. Learning to trust your body will provide the freedom and beauty you desire to experience in this remarkable life.

Your body is intelligent and has the complete ability to heal itself. Think about the last time you got a cut. Your body was capable of stopping the bleeding, scabbing, and healing that cut all on its own. You may have covered it with a band-aid to help, but it was *your body* that created new cells and put you back together. Whenever you're sick, your body knows just what to do to help you get back to where your body is happy, healthy, and comfortable. Our bodies are capable of things beyond what our minds can comprehend. Your job is learning to trust your intelligent body. The more you can get in tune with your body, the more at ease you'll feel in your skin. And, just like changing a band-aid, replacing old limiting beliefs with new, empowering ones will help your wounds begin to heal.

The diet mindset instructs women to listen to the

celeb weight loss expert or follow the hot social media influencer to teach them how to get healthy and happy, but the truth is that you don't need someone encouraging you to eat as they do. You don't need someone to tell you what is right and wrong for your body because it's likely that you already know. The key to discovering it is to stop listening to the outside noise and focus on yourself. Pay attention to what food makes you feel the most energized, what food makes you feel good about yourself, and which foods nourish you in different ways. Your body can tell you all of that if you ask yourself the right questions and trust that your body will give you the answers.

Your body communicates. It tells you what it needs to heal and thrive; you just need to cultivate silence and start listening. When you experience a symptom like a stomachache, headache, or back pain, your body is communicating there is an imbalance. I've come to realize whenever I get a stiff neck, my body is silently begging for more rest from screens. I've learned what makes my body feel its best requires reflecting on the feedback and taking action to change it. Just like at work when your boss gives you feedback or at home when a partner gives you feedback, you don't ignore them. You listen and change your habits to be better for the relationships you value—and the relationship with your body should be no different. Take a darn minute, turn off your busy monkey brain, and listen to what your body is trying to tell you.

Another way our body communicates to us is through our emotions. Have you ever needed to let yourself cry? Like, full-on waterworks, snot, and noise that lies somewhere between a hungry piglet and angry cat? The kind of cry that makes you bury your face in a pillow, so no one has the chance of getting a peek at your crying face. If so, you know this sort of cry is likely accompanied by actual heart pain or a dreadful knot in your stomach. Yet the more you allow yourself to heave and let the sadness pour out of you, the tears slow, and the sadness ceases. One can only describe this kind of cry as cathartic, and afterward, one feels better and physically lighter.

Our emotions are energy running through our body, and it's another way our body communicates to us what we might need. When you feel anxious, stressed, or overwhelmed, perhaps your body is asking to be grounded in the present moment by going for a walk or meditating on your breath. When your temper flares and you feel frustrated and angry, maybe it's a signal from your body that you need to release some stress by punching a pillow or lifting weights at the gym. Take the feelings that come up and sit in them. Feel them instead of ignoring them and pushing them away. Connect your mind to your body. Then, ask yourself what you need to do at the moment to feel more grounded, more joyful, and more relaxed, and I guarantee you will be able to come up with an answer. There are times when you might need to suppress emotions, like while we're at work, but it's important to find a way to release them so those emotions don't stay trapped in your body.

Emotions give us insight into ourselves if we choose to listen. Part of trusting your body is allowing emotions to pass through you and try to find out what they are trying to communicate. You are not your emotions; they are simply energy passing through your body. Emotions come and go, but you remain. There is no need to try and label our feelings as ours. When you say things like "I am sad," you are identifying sadness as part of your identity. Instead, say, "I'm experiencing sadness right now," or "A feeling of sadness is passing through me." Be impeccable with your word, as Don Miguel, the author of *The Four Agreements*, instructs.[1] Allowing emotional clearance is essential for well-being. The more you allow your cooped-up energy to be released, the more space you create for the positive emotions of joy, gratitude, and abundance. Not to mention you will feel lighter and develop a more positive, loving relationship with your brilliant body.

Trusting your body also means giving it what it needs to thrive in this empowered life outside the cave you are creating for yourself. Your body needs nutrients from whole foods which are the foundational building blocks to help your body function at its best. When you focus your energy on eating well, the topic just covered in the previous chapter, you will start to notice how much better you feel. Your mood improves, and your thinking gets clearer. You experience higher, sustained energy levels throughout your day. The more you focus on nourishing yourself over restricting yourself, you will feel stronger while also feeling lighter. When you take care of your body, your body begins to take care of you right back. Wholesome nutrition, joyful movement, adequate sleep, and proactive stress management will help your body thrive while also improving your mental and emotional health. You won't have to feel as though you're fighting against your body because you are learning to work alongside it.

If you're reading this and biting your nails, overwhelmed at the idea of trusting your body, you're certainly not alone. Many patients that I've seen throughout the years have felt the apprehension that comes with stepping outside of the cave and into a whole new world. We as humans like to stay within the boundary of our comfort zones because we feel safe and secure in our bubble. But, girl, you will never have true freedom if you stay locked in the cave. Close your eyes and envision your happiest and healthiest self again right now. She is not worried about *how* she will embody happiness and health, but she does—mastering the health mindset will show you *how* to make it happen without needing logic, reasoning, or conscious thought. That is really the goal of this book. To make the health mindset an ingrained part of who you are so that thinking empowering thoughts, making conscious emotional choices instead of reacting, and engaging in health-focused behaviors becomes genuinely part of who you are. It won't be something you *need* to do, but just another part of *who you are*. Putting your faith into the health mindset and your body will guide you to transform.

Get in tune with the natural rhythms of your body. As you practice mindfulness while you're eating, listen to the cues that your body gives you. What does your body feel like when it's hungry? What are the warning signs it gives you when you've gone too long without eating? How does your body respond after a well-balanced meal in comparison to a wimpy salad that a rabbit wouldn't even eat? Paying attention to your hunger cues is an important part of listening to your body and trusting that you are giving her what she needs. For so long, women have denied themselves food when they are truly hungry, only to result in ravenous, uncontrollable hunger.

As a dietitian, I hear it all the time from the patient who only eats a piece of fruit and coffee for breakfast and wonders why she doesn't have any energy to the patient who chews gum and drinks a gallon of water to fend off hunger pangs because she already exceeded her calories for the day. When you are so used to denying your body what it needs, it might feel foreign to begin to actually listen to it. Feelings of discomfort are normal. Your body tends to know what you need before your mind does, and it's important to get in tune with your eating rhythms and cues from your body in order to start giving it the nourishment it needs.

On the flip side, getting to know your satiation cues is equally as important. What does your body say when you forcefully overeat because you were programmed to clean your plate? How does your body respond when you snack mindlessly to forget about a crappy day? Eating mindfully helps to make sure you are consciously eating and allows you to listen to your body while fueling it. You don't need to finish your entire plate of food if you're full. You don't have to eat food that others prepare when you know the food won't help you to feel your best. Getting to know what your body needs and craves helps you to get to know what your body is trying to communicate and how much food is truly enough. When you don't take the time to learn what your body feels like once it's had enough, you may continue to struggle with your nutrition. It's normal to overeat sometimes, but it shouldn't be a regular occurrence. Getting to know your satiety cues will help you to learn the difference between feeling full and comfortable versus feeling stuffed and uncomfortable. It takes time and practice to begin getting comfortable with the cues your body gives you and learning how to respect them. Sometimes simple shifts like eating more mindfully, slowing down to take sips of a drink, or chewing your food a bit more can help your body catch up to the food that you're eating. It's not about restricting your food or about limiting the amount you eat. It's really about learning for yourself when you've reached the right fullness instead of blindly eating past the point of comfort.

This is where I tend to get the question from patients: *But will this help me lose weight?* This question is a tough one, but I always give my patients the same answer; maybe. If weight loss is part of your healthiest self, adopting a health mindset might help your weight trend down naturally. I've had patients who barely tipped the scale, but their bodies drastically transformed. They lost inches around their waist and reported feeling lighter with more energy. This is a better representation of health than a silly little number on the scale.

Many people are desperate to lose weight, but desperation typically originates from a 'lack' mindset. Women, in particular, feel like they have to lose weight right now, or for a wedding in a week, or summer in a month, and it pushes them to extremes. If weight loss is important to your healthiest self, it's important to lose weight with patience and self-compassion. Trust that your body knows what is best and that when you lose weight in a slow and sustainable way, you're more likely to keep the weight and inches off for good. Wouldn't you rather take a few months or a year to lose weight but keep it off for the remainder of your life than constantly starve yourself for weeks at a time, only to gain back all the weight you lost plus some? Trust your body and be grateful for how amazing she is and how well she takes care of you. The more trust you can place in your body and listen to the feedback it gives you, the better you will consistently feel, and whatever weight you want to lose will naturally fall away.

Release the need to have all the answers for yourself right now. Many patients I've worked with get caught up in *how* they will lose weight if that is a part of their happiest and healthiest self. They demand to know *how* to make it happen and want a concrete plan with rules and definitive steps to follow. That's what makes the health mindset different from the diet mindset. The *how* is not something that will be definitively outlined for you here because *how* will look different for every person. The diet mindset prescribes hard rules everyone must follow in order to reach one specific goal and, as we already discussed at length, that one goal might not be the same goal that you have. Dietary dogma interrupts personalized nutrition.

Eating well is not cookie cutter. The health mindset takes into account *your* definition of health and *your* health and nutrition goals. To reach our different goals, one person might adjust their food to be more nutrient-based while another person might start including more movement throughout their day. Once the health mindset is mastered, the *how* will present itself for each person.

9

THE NEVER-ENDING STORY

Your health and happiness are not a destination to be reached but rather a journey you commit yourself to. Health and happiness are a conscious choice you make every single day and not a place that you end up and can camp out at. There is no definitive end to health and happiness because they are a state of mind and a state of being. Because we have the privilege of being human, it means we also have the wild roller coaster of emotions and a plethora of reasons *not* to focus on health and joy. There will always be occurrences that threaten your happiness and health, which is why taking control of your well-being is not a simple, one-time fix. The health mindset is a foundation that you build over your life. It is a choice we make day in and day out because we are worthy of love and joy, and freedom. I wish change could happen overnight, but the truth is that change requires patience, self-compassion, and trust in yourself.

I remember back when I was living with a dieter's mindset. I was trapped by the rules of the diet culturescape and lived my life bound in chains of inadequacy. The drive to eat well was never self-love but self-rejection. I never thought I was good enough the way I was. Thin was never thin enough. I knew I could have a better body. Before every vacation, a restrictive diet ushered in because I didn't believe my body was good enough to sit on a sunny beach unless I had abs. Looking back now, it was punishment working myself to the bone so I could enjoy a week on a beautiful beach. Even with my strict diet, I would still feel the urge to cover my stomach for fear that it still wasn't good enough.

After years of studying self-love and nutrition, my habit of dieting before vacationing disappeared. I didn't just wake up one day feeling as though I was ready to accept my body as it was, but it was a careful and thoughtful shift that happened day after day, week after week until I felt comfortable and confident in my own skin. I remember the first vacation where I felt no desire to restrict myself the week before. Let me tell you; the results were joyous. I felt truly free for the first time in a very long time. I felt safe and secure in my body to show up exactly as I was. I felt comfortable in my body and at ease with my thoughts, emotions, and actions. It was the first time that I wanted to run and play while at the beach instead of laying on a towel, desperately tanning because darker skin made me appear skinnier. Or praying my body didn't jiggle as I ran into the water. I wasn't obsessed with the way my bathing suit fit or concerned about what other people thought of the cellulite on my legs or whether or not my belly folded when I sat down. I enjoyed the beach and my time there with my full heart, feeling incredibly grateful for my experience. I thought since I achieved body freedom on this trip, and many others after, I was totally free. But the liar is always waiting for the one vulnerable moment it can chime in.

Recently, I went on a vacation to Hawaii. The days leading up to the trip had been the most self-loved, fueled days of my life. I felt joyful and confident in my body and my relationship with food. I didn't feel the urge to diet before the trip and allowed myself to feel worthy of the incredible vacation that awaited me. My sister blessed us with an incredible and luxurious resort. Just when I thought my self-love was the strongest it had ever been, all the positive energy flew out the window when we landed at the resort. Here I was, at a gorgeous resort surrounded by gorgeous people. Women with tall, slender bodies and flawless skin walked past me. I was instantly triggered and found myself looking down at my short body and feeling ashamed. My old conditioning and limiting beliefs began swirling around my head.

> *I can't believe I didn't even try to diet for this trip. I literally teach people how to eat for a living . . . why did I have to eat so many d*mn brownies last weekend? How did I not even try to get a few extra workouts in, so my stomach looks a little flatter and toned before coming here? You don't deserve to be here because you're not as rich, beautiful, and slender as the other women. You are a fraud.*

These negative thoughts began popping up one after another, causing me to feel terrible about myself and my body. Because I have worked on self-love and empowerment for so long, I had the ability to step back into my awareness throne, take a deep breath, and observe these negative thoughts and emotions before they could take root in my mind. Instead of giving into these limiting thoughts and having a terrible time the remainder of my trip, feeling shame about my "imperfect" body, I simply acknowledged the thoughts and feelings that were coming up. I remembered the old limiting beliefs my younger self used to believe. But I didn't let the liar win. I said out loud and to myself, "*I choose to love my beautiful, amazing body the way she is right now. I am free and I am happy.*" I repeated this mantra the entire trip and accepted this vulnerable moment as a test. I practiced loving my beautiful body anyways. The health mindset is not a quick fix, and maintaining the foundation requires patience, love, and kindness because health is a never-ending story.

Adopting a health mindset means knowing and understanding that old conditioning will flare up. Having a health mindset doesn't mean you will never struggle with negative, self-deprecating thoughts again, but instead gives you the awareness to exercise power and control over what beliefs you endorse. Observe the thought instead of aligning with it. It's in your awareness power that you can say, "*Oh, look how I just beat myself up there.*" It's your responsibility to stop playing the depressing movie in your head.

While I know some people will feel like they *need* to have the liar in their head to succeed, I will agree to disagree. You can't shame yourself into making a change. And you definitely can't hate yourself into a version of yourself you can love.

Some things make adopting a health mindset easier, and one of those things is eliminating triggers. At the beginning of your mind transformation, cleaning up your surroundings is essential. When you find yourself triggered by old dieter's mindset beliefs, which you likely will, it's important to go back to the basics. Try to understand how and where these thoughts originated and developed. Ask yourself if these beliefs are truth or lies. Are they coming from a place of loving your magnificent body or from the pressures and expectations of society to eat a certain way or weigh a certain amount? Remember that this unconscious programming is not your fault, but in order to outgrow the dieter's mindset cave, you must take responsibility for them. It's imperative you become aware of these limiting beliefs and begin to notice how they might be impacting you and keeping you small.

One reason the dieter's mindset is so pervasive is because it is borne from its own toxic culture that permeates every nook and cranny of society. Your friends and family members are likely deep in the dieter's cave without really knowing it. Women are constantly bombarded with messaging and images that scream at us, telling us that our bodies are wrong and bad unless we are thin. The diet culturescape teaches women that if they are not thin, then they are not metabolically healthy, and this messaging leads women to adopt a strict dieter's mindset. The dieter's mindset is riddled with limiting beliefs that keep women stuck in repeating the same disempowering behaviors, unhealthful emotions, and negative thoughts when it comes to food and their bodies. The limiting beliefs persist in many different areas and in a variety of ways that actually harm health rather than help women achieve health. If you notice that the people you love, friends and family, are stuck in this state of mind, it's okay to refuse to engage in the conversations around body, food, and diet. Allow yourself permission to set boundaries around the sorts of conversations you want to engage in.

I'm sure you've heard the cliche saying, "You are the average of the five people you spend the most time with." It's a universal truth! Notice how your friends and family talk about food and their bodies. Do they use empowered language, or do they speak from a set of limiting beliefs that you no longer prescribe to? Whenever I am talking with a non-patient who clearly has a dieter's mindset and insists on talking about their "bad" foods or "terrible, fat body," I simply listen and then change the topic of conversation. It's not your job to try and free everyone from the cave. Each prisoner must free herself. But you can set boundaries, so you do not get sucked into the negative spiral. Be the light, and they may eventually follow.

If the people around you aren't supportive, find

other like-minded people you can surround yourself with. Join an online support group with others who are rewriting their definition of health and cultivating a better relationship with their body and food. Hire a coach or a therapist who can validate your feelings and continue to empower you to work on your limiting beliefs. Start reaching out to new circles of people who are actively trying to work on improving themselves and see how you can get involved with them. When you're surrounded by empowered and uplifting people, you are more likely to feel the same. Community comes in handy when you feel as though you need accountability; you have a whole group of potential check-in partners! Don't be afraid to go outside of your comfort zone to find other women who are on a similar journey and who can be cheerleaders and mentors as you start your health mindset journey.

You might not be able to get rid of a toxic family member, so another trigger eliminator is cleaning up your social media. Sadly, there are way too many accounts on social media that encourage a dieter's mindset or use their platforms to perpetuate diet myths. The more you can distance yourself from those pandering a diet mindset, the better you will feel.

I don't know why I used to follow women who

were much taller than me for inspiration; I'm 5' 1" and no matter what exercise I do or foods I eat, I am not getting any taller. I found it helpful to replace those old "fitspo" accounts with women who weren't obsessed with their looks. I discovered intellectual women who celebrate individuality, character, and health over a bubble butt, perky boobs, and perfect eyebrows, lips, and face. If a perfect body triggers your ego, it might be a good idea to temporarily unfollow them while you are building your health foundation.

Once you start becoming aware of the diet culturescape, you'll realize it's everywhere. It's up to you to decide what you believe and to choose more empowering thoughts and engage with other empowered people. Remember that replacing beliefs is done through conscious practice and compassion. Bringing awareness to your limiting beliefs is the first step. You are allowed to leave behind the thoughts, emotions, and behaviors that no longer serve you. The things that helped you as a kid are not necessarily the same things that will help you as an adult. Remember your values and use the tools of intentionality. Use journaling to create space for novel thoughts, recite your affirmations, practice gratitude to increase positive emotional energy, meditate to quiet the mind to connect with your true self, and visualize and embody your highest self.

Rewiring beliefs comes down to thinking different thoughts and doing things in a different way. Both of these things take conscious effort and patience with yourself so you can give your focus and energy to the things that empower you instead of the things that make you feel ashamed or a failure. Prove to yourself that the limiting beliefs you hold are false. Grab a pen and your favorite journal to start writing about them. Just write down what you can remember about how these beliefs may have begun or when they started popping up for clarity around them. Acknowledge that these beliefs have worked to keep you safe for a long time but also understand that these limiting beliefs are not your truth.

Reconnect with yourself often. I find that many patients I have are committed to their health mindset when things are otherwise going well in their life. It's harder to commit to the health mindset when you're under copious amounts of stress. You might find yourself focusing on thoughts and emotions that don't align with your values or make you feel empowered. The way to combat this is by connecting with yourself as often as you can. Some patients of mine do this on Sunday evenings, while others do it first thing on Monday mornings. Still, some commit to it every morning. Rehearse your definition of health and decide what aspect of health you are going to embody during the week ahead. Set an intention to drive your behavior. An intention can simply be a word or short phrase such as "self-respect" or "I choose to eat well to nourish my body." This keeps you connected to your personal mission for health and helps to drown out the noise that does not represent your authentic voice and your empowering truth.

Connecting with yourself often helps keep you motivated to make empowering choices. The best and easiest way to connect with yourself is to imagine your happiest and healthiest self as often as you can. Feel the feelings as if you were embodying her right now. A study done in 1991 explored the connection between visualizing and the brain to find that mental rehearsal (specifically, visualization) of events enhanced performance on cognitive tasks.[1] When you visualize yourself living your happiest and healthiest life, your brain is strengthening the connections of your empowering beliefs, which means you have less resistance to aligning your life with them. By consciously connecting with the person you aspire to be and aligning yourself with her as much as possible, you will inevitably create stories, thoughts, and emotions that are empowering you to take action on your health. When you visualize your best self, don't just visualize the way she acts but also the way she thinks, takes care of herself, and expresses her emotions. Practicing putting yourself in her shoes will help align with her every day and allow you to stay focused on your new beliefs about health instead of limiting ones.

Eating well and a health mindset require you to get to know your body and to improve the relationship you have with your food by consciously connecting with yourself over and over again. As you learn to eat well, it's imperative to practice mindful eating. Use all your senses to feel into your meals. Slow down and experience every part of the food that you're eating. Eating well also means being thankful and having gratitude for the food you eat and the body that digests the meal. Eating well asks women to listen to their own body to decide what it needs and trusting that their body will tell them when it needs something different. Listen to your body's hunger cues and satiation cues. What does your body feel like when it's peckish, hungry, and starving? What does your body feel like when it's full or overstuffed? Getting comfortable with the process of slowing down and bringing awareness to your body will only help you learn how to fuel your body with both nutritious foods and treats that contribute to a happy and healthy body and mind.

Eating well requires you to have faith in your body and to place trust in your food choices. Trust that your body knows how to heal itself and that it will tell you when it needs more or when you've had enough. Trust that you can live a life that is happy and healthy without the restriction and shame of the dieter's mindset. Also, know that trusting yourself and your body means letting go of fear for courageous eating.

The dieter's mindset asks women to ignore their body signals to eat six small meals a day, eat 1,200 calorie diets, or use food restriction as a punishment for feeding themselves. None of these teach women how to eat well but simply teach them how to eat less. Eating and weighing less is not necessarily what is best. This is why having a reference to your own definition of health is so important. This is why a health mindset will actually help you become a healthier person. You don't need to prescribe to these extreme limitations to be healthy, which is why trusting your body and aligning yourself with your definition of health and your empowering beliefs are the best thing you can do to embody a health mindset.

I stopped making "to-do" lists regarding my

health a while ago. If I didn't check everything off my list, I felt like a failure. Also, I wasted precious time writing the same things over and over again. *Exercise, journal, book write, cook, meditate, write some more, read, work… blah blah blah.* It was a list that made me feel overwhelmed from just looking at it. So, I abandoned the habit of making a checklist and adopted the practice of being in the present moment. Now, I just picture my healthiest self and embody her. This quick visualization saves a lot of time when I would typically spend hours a week thinking about "what do I need to do?" Nowadays, it's easy and natural for me to work out four days a week without any resistance.

You don't need to make a checklist, but you need to check in with yourself regularly. Every morning I start my day by asking myself how I'm feeling and what my highest self would do. Sometimes this means I rest. Other times it means I move my body in the sunshine, while other times, I need to dance in my bathroom while I get ready for work. Checking in with myself means I can prioritize my day based on my needs alone, and it allows me to make healthy choices all day—even when that may mean having some ice cream with my husband or skipping a gym workout in favor of gardening in the sunshine. It allows me to make choices that align with what I need to support my health that day. Reconnecting with your highest self every morning keeps her characteristics fresh in your head, so you focus on empowering choices instead of fear and limitation that exists everywhere in the diet culturescape.

Remember, change is inevitable. We, just like the seasons and amount of sunlight, change all the time. We go through periods of dormancy and periods of rapid growth. We go through bountiful harvests and seasons where it rains all the time. Change is the only thing that is constant throughout our lives, and yet it is the thing we fear the most. Get comfortable with change. Make friends with it and with the incredible world that is waiting for you outside the cave. You may find a new appreciation and love for nourishing foods. You may also begin to enjoy treats that you haven't allowed yourself to enjoy for most of your life and realize that enjoying those foods intentionally and in moderation *doesn't* make you gain weight. Accepting that change is a part of life will help you realize that what you eat today may not be what you need to eat tomorrow for your physical and emotional health. You allow yourself periods of life that your health centers around eating well, while in other weeks, your health focuses on enjoyable movement. Allow yourself to grow and change to experience life to the fullest. You were never meant to stay the same.

You were never meant to waste your precious time in life trying to perpetually make yourself smaller. Take up space, live at full volume, and live the life of joy and health that you've always wanted because it is available to you now.

There is also no shame in asking for help. One area of the diet mindset that persists within people is if they aren't meeting their goals, they alone are to blame. This leaves women thinking and feeling that if they just had more self-control, or if they were just a little more disciplined, they could have great health and a better body. But this is not the case. Rewiring limiting beliefs is hard work, and no one expects you to be able to do it all on your own. It's okay to ask for help or support. If you need more guidance on uprooting your limiting beliefs or if the journey gets too uncomfortable to manage on your own, I recommend working with a dietitian or a therapist who can gently guide your awareness to help shift your belief system. You might find that one limiting belief is incredibly easy for you to shift, but others are much more stubborn. This is not a reflection on you, how hard you're trying, or how badly you want to get healthy. It is simply information that you and a professional can use to help walk away from disempowering beliefs in order to help you create new, more empowering beliefs.

Mastering a health mindset will be a different journey for every person, but it will still be a journey. Just when you think you've cleared out all your limiting beliefs, you may find a new one. Limiting beliefs are something every single person on this planet deals with, from supermodels on a catwalk to your next-door neighbor. You can't expect to have the same results as the person next to you because your mind, body, and soul are vastly different. Working on a health mindset is an investment in yourself. It's an investment in your health and your longevity. It's never too late for you to radically transform your belief system. It is not too late for you to experience health and joy. All it takes is the decision to commit to yourself and take one small step forward daily, and you will reap the benefits that unfold over time.

Understand that a health mindset is not a destination you arrive at but something you will perpetually work on. The diet culturescape exists everywhere you look: social media, magazine covers, and movies. It can be difficult to rewire the dieter's mindset because the limiting beliefs contained within it can be found anywhere and everywhere, down to your laundry detergent ads. Knowing that the dieter's mindset may never go away will help you anticipate the limiting beliefs that inevitably pop up over time.

The health mindset is a never-ending story that

encourages you to make the conscious choice to align yourself with the health mindset every day. Changes happen in small ways over time and with practice. You will have a health mindset and the freedom that comes along with it the minute you decide to start feeding yourself empowering beliefs, thoughts, emotions, and actions. But you earn a health mindset by choosing those things every day by visualizing your happiest, healthiest self. By connecting with yourself and your definition of health every day. By embodying the happiest and healthiest version of you every single day.

The health mindset is not a quick fix to health and happiness. It is a conscious rewiring from the painful limits of the past so that you can create the future of your dreams. While integrating a health mindset can take time, you can decide right now that you are done living in the dieter's cave. Decide right now that your health and happiness are not reserved for a version of you that is thin but for you as you exist in this very moment. You have the power in your hands to live the life you want. You will never achieve it if you don't first believe it. What is stopping you from believing in your inevitable health, happiness, and success today? It's only you and the fear about exiting the comfortable cave. You can choose to stay stuck in the darkness of the cave and forever fear the world outside of it, or you can choose to see things in a different light. The choice, the power, the health, and the happiness are yours for the taking as soon as you say *yes* to yourself. You have all the tools and resources required for your success inside you. Now it's time to go out and use them!

NEXT STEPS FOR YOUR HEALTH JOURNEY

Are you ready to take the next step to eating well?

Learn more about the Longevity Nutrition in

Hungry for Truth: Ditch the Lies About Dieting and Discover the Truth About Longevity Nutrition in a World of Misinformation

Available in print and ebook form on Amazon.

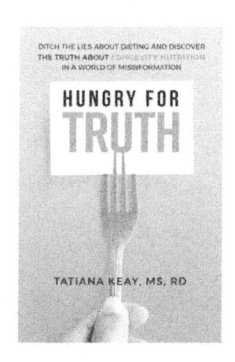

Longevity Nutrition is the closest natural thing we have to the Fountain of Youth. Eat well, age gracefully, and live your one life to the fullest.

Join the Community

Join Well-Being with Dietitian Tatiana on Facebook to take part in a community of health-conscious individuals. This is a safe and optimistic place to ask questions about nutrition, health, and mindset.

Your Voice Matters

If you loved this book, please leave a review on Amazon. I love reading each and every review! Your feedback helps me create more useful content for you in the future. (It also really helps newer authors!) You may also email me your thoughts and feedback at dietitiantatiana@gmail.com.

Stay in Touch

www.vitaminkeay.com
Instagram: @VitaminKeayRD
Tag me in your stories/posts so I can repost!

ACKNOWLEDGMENTS

Thank you to my anchor and safe haven, Colby, who has shown me unconditional love, even on my off days.

Thank you to my family for believing in me and encouraging me to be my best self.

Thank you to my best friends for being there when I felt like I was walking on a tightrope about to fall.

Thank you to my publishing team: Lauren, Johanna, and Sampath, for helping me create this book.

And a special thank you to all my patients who have taught me more about the human mind and eating behaviors than a textbook alone.

Finally, thank you to God for giving me the ability to create and experience this life. And thank you to Jesus for being the perfect example – may I continue to strive to be like You.

My gift to you!

For more support on your health journey, here is your free downloadable weight loss guide.

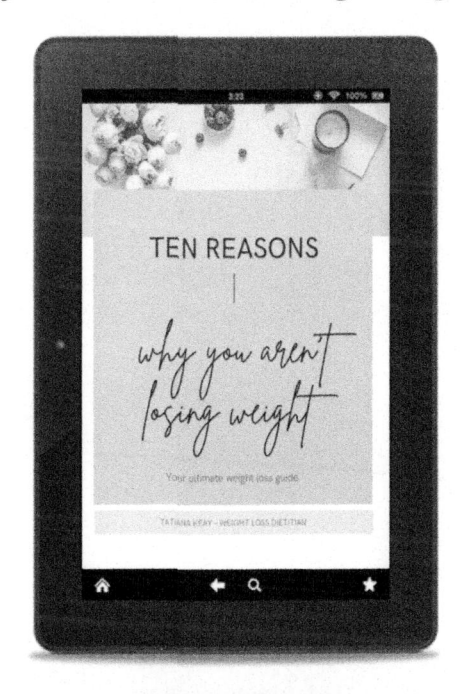

http://freeguide.vitaminkeay.com/

NOTES

2. The Dieter's Mindset

1. Kopala-Sibley, D. C., Zuroff, D. C., Hankin, B. L., & Abela, J. R. Z. (2015). The Development of Self-Criticism and Dependency in Early Adolescence and Their Role in the Development of Depressive and Anxiety Symptoms. *Personality and Social Psychology Bulletin*, *41*(8), 1094–1109. https://doi.org/10.1177/0146167215590985.
2. Fardouly, J., & Vartanian, L. R. (2015). Negative Comparisons about one's appearance Mediate the relationship between Facebook Usage and body Image concerns. *Body Image, 12*(), 82–88. https://doi.org/10.1016/j.bodyim.2014.10.004.

3. The Health Mindset

1. Dunaev, J., Markey, C. H., & Brochu, P. M. (2018). An attitude of gratitude: The effects of body-focused gratitude on weight bias internalization and body image. *Body Image, 25*, 9–13. https://doi.org/10.1016/j.bodyim.2018.01.006.
2. Roberts, C. J., Campbell, I. C., & Troop, N. (2013). Increases in Weight during Chronic Stress are Partially Associated with a Switch in Food Choice towards Increased Carbohydrate and Saturated Fat Intake. *European Eating Disorders Review, 22*(1), 77–82. https://doi.org/10.1002/erv.2264

4. Awareness

1. Vaish, A., Grossmann, T., & Woodward, A. (2008). Not all emotions are created equal: The negativity bias in social-emotional development. *Psychological Bulletin, 134*(3), 383–403. https://doi.org/10.1037/00332909.134.3.383.
2. Rounsefell, K., Gibson, S., McLean, S., Blair, M., Molenaar, A., Brennan, L., Truby, H., & McCaffrey, T. A. (2019). Social media, body image and food choices in healthy young adults: A mixed methods systematic review. *Nutrition & Dietetics, 77*(1). https://doi.org/10.1111/1747-0080.12581.

5. Rewiring Your Beliefs

1. Dr. Caroline Leaf. (2019, May 9). *Why We Keep Making the Same Mistakes + Tips to Break Bad Habits*. Dr. Leaf; Dr. Leaf. https://drleaf.com/blogs/news/why-we-keep-making-the-same-mistakes-tips-to-break-bad-habits.
2. Dunaev, J., Markey, C. H., & Brochu, P. M. (2018). An attitude of gratitude: The effects of body-focused gratitude on weight bias internalization and body image. *Body Image, 25*, 9–13. https://doi.org/10.1016/j.bodyim.2018.01.006.
3. Fritz, M. M., Armenta, C. N., Walsh, L. C., & Lyubomirsky, S. (2019). Gratitude facilitates healthy eating behavior in adolescents and young adults. *Journal of Experimental Social Psychology, 81*, 4–14. https://doi.org/10.1016/j.jesp.2018.08.011.

6. Rewrite Your Definition of Health

1. Zhang, Z., Chen, W. A Systematic Review of the Relationship Between Physical Activity and Happiness. *J Happiness Stud* **20,** 1305–1322 (2019). https://doi.org/10.1007/s10902-018-9976-0.

8. Trust Your Body Temple

1. Don Miguel Ruiz. (2008). *The Four Agreements*. Hay House Inc.

9. The Never-Ending Story

1. Ungerleider, S., & Golding, J. M. (1991). Mental Practice among Olympic Athletes. *Perceptual and Motor Skills*, *72*(3), 1007–1017. https://doi.org/10.2466/pms.1991.72.3.1007.

Printed in Great Britain
by Amazon